YOUR YOGA BIRTHGUIDE

JENNY BEEKEN

Jenny has been teaching yoga to pregnant women for nearly thirty years and seen them flourish and bloom through their practice. With her colleague Pauline Sawyer she has established the Inner Yoga Trust and Inner Yoga School to train teachers in yoga awareness.

Jenny met Sally Townsend shortly before becoming pregnant with her daughter, Beth, who was born in 1989. Sally was practising as an independent midwife and Jenny asked Sally to attend her through her pregnancy. Sally was herself pregnant with her own daughter Alice and the two women helped each other through the postnatal period and with the raising of a young family. A firm and lasting friendship developed.

At this time Jenny ran ante- and postnatal classes with a crèche. They were lovely relaxed classes, where the babies came in and out to be fed and the toddlers knew their mother was just close by if needed. The classes gave mothers time to balance and restore their energies.

When Jenny decided to develop the pregnancy module for the Inner Yoga School it seemed natural to ask Sally to collaborate, and thus arose the urge to create a book that would act as a reference for midwives wanting to integrate yoga into their professional lives, for yoga teachers needing a reference to aid their teaching, and for pregnant women wanting to continue their yoga practice through pregnancy.

SALLY TOWNSEND

Sally Townsend was a Registered Midwife for over twenty years before her death in May 2008, and during this time personally delivered over a hundred and seventy babies. This book is now dedicated to her memory, her wonderful skills as a midwife, a teacher and a dear friend who is missed every day, especially in the completion of this book.

Sally developed and ran the first pregnancy module for the Inner Yoga School alongside Jenny in 2006/7. She brought to the Inner Yoga Trust's courses an in-depth experience and comprehensive knowledge of the anatomy and physiology of the mother and baby during pregnancy, birth and the postnatal period. She advised a wide range of women on all aspects of pregnancy and birth, and in this book she offers you an awareness and understanding of the changes that pregnancy brings, so that you can best understand what are the most suitable yoga postures and movements.

Sally practised yoga herself for most of her life, albeit spasmodically! She shows full awareness of the benefits yoga can give to everybody, but specifically to the pregnant and postnatal woman. Her family have all been involved one way or another in the publication of this book, as have several of Sally's former colleagues. Her son Patrick had the challenging task of the photo retouching, so that the combination of professional and amateur photographs complement each other.

OTHER BOOKS BY JENNY BEEKEN

YOGA OF THE HEART : A WHITE EAGLE BOOK OF YOGA
YOUR YOGA BODYMAP FOR VITALITY
DON'T HOLD YOUR BREATH
ANCIENT WISDOM

Your Yoga Birthguide

JENNY BEEKEN AND SALLY TOWNSEND

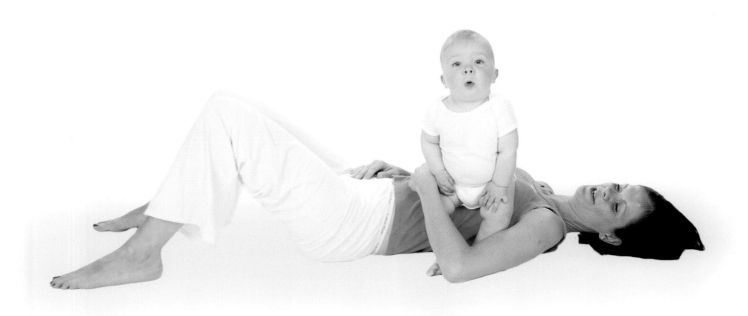

POLAIR PUBLISHING ▪ LONDON

First published November 2009
by Polair Publishing, P O Box 34886
London W8 6YR
Distributed in the USA and Canada by SCB Distributors

British Library Cataloguing-in-Publication Data
A catalogue record for this book is available from the British Library
ISBN 978-1-905398-19-5

The information provided in this book is based on information available at the time of publication but should not be construed as substitute for personal medical advice or instruction. Yoga and midwifery practitioners should have regard to any information on these matters which may become available subsequent to the preparation of this book, and no action on the part of individuals should be taken based solely on the contents of this book. Readers should consult appropriate health professionals on any matter relating to their health and wellbeing. The information and opinions provided here are believed to be accurate and sound, based on the best judgment available to the authors, but readers who fail to consult appropriate health authorities assume the risk of any injuries.

Set in Century Gothic and
and printed in Great Britain by
Cambridge University Press

CONTENTS

LIST OF DIAGRAMS

ACKNOWLEDGMENTS

Acknowledgments and thanks are due to the photographers Michael Prior, Michael Stone, Sue Peggs, Alice Snel
de Gans, Dawn Baillie, Daryl Hedley, Patrick Townsend and Julian Warde, and especially to Patrick for his studio work on the
photographs; also to Rosemary Young for producing the anatomical drawings. My thanks also to Donna Ockenden, Pauline
Sawyer, Fiona Bruce, Joy Hosie, Marielle Churaqui, Will Lane, Janis Binnie and Dawn Baillie for their advice and contributions,
and additionally to Fiona for her editing and care in the final stages. My sincere thanks to Charlie Hartley for her diligence
and great care and awareness in editing and indexing. Charles Townsend and Clare Fletcher have given great support
and I thank them. I am grateful to Colum Hayward, at Polair Publishing, who has been extremely supportive,
understanding and caring in the journey this book has been on in the last eighteen months.
Lastly, thanks to my daughter Beth (Elizabeth Grace, meaning a gift from God)
for being the greatest teacher to me on my life path.

*I am grateful to the authors and publishers of the copyright works from which brief extract has been made, namely Newmarket Press,
Dr Francis Leboyer and Sri BKS Iyengar for the extract from INNER BEAUTY, INNER LIGHT on p. 52; to HarperCollins and Alastair Shearer and Peter
Russell for the words from the Chhandogya Upanishad on pp. 72 and 109 and to Rider & Co and Alistair Shearer for the quotation from
Patanjali on p. 89; to HarperCollins and the estate of Vanda Scaravelli for the quotations from AWAKENING THE SPINE on pp. 96 and 120; to Hands
on Health and Victor van Kooten for the quotation from FROM INSIDE OUT on p. 99; to Judith O'Reilly for words from her blog 'Wife in the North'
quoted on p. 102, and to Penguin Books and Eckhardt Tolle for the quotation from A NEW EARTH on p. 119.*

All the world's a stage
And all the men and women merely players;
They have their exits and their entrances,
And one man in his time plays many parts,
His acts being seven ages. At first the infant,
Mewling and puking in the nurse's arms.
And then the whining schoolboy....
Shakespeare, *As You Like It*

Introduction

 PREGNANCY is a vitally important, wonderful, sometimes fearful time in a woman's life; a time that needs space, respect, great care and attention.

It requires us to come out of our day-to-day existence and be totally aware of this wonderful event that is taking place.

We need time and space to do this, and support and understanding from those close to us and from those in the professions that help women through this time. In YOUR YOGA BIRTHGUIDE, we have sought to offer a combination of the yoga teacher's support and advice with the more technical assistance a midwife brings, which we hope will increase the level of support the mother can have at this time.

We have all sorts of feelings during our pregnancy, from not wanting the process at all (or at least at this time in our life!) through to being overjoyed with expectation. Yoga and meditation can give us space to be thrilled and clarity to consider any important decisions that need to be made, so that we are less likely to be over-influenced by others or thrown into turmoil by their advice. The decisions need to be ours, and our partner's, throughout. The father of the baby may have different views from ours. The practice of yoga and meditation together can bring more understanding and harmony to what is happening – and what is going to happen or needs to happen.

There can also be feelings of fear. Our bodies are taken over and 'run' by this coming event of birth, especially after we have been through the first trimester (three-month period). Fear and anticipation of the birth itself and all that it entails is understandable, but yoga enables us to have more control and awareness.

We feel our body changing, and we wonder if it will ever recover. I remember one friend saying, 'I know how the baby got in there but how on earth is it going to get out?'! This is a surprisingly common feeling. A huge concern is that our baby should be healthy, normal, happy. About this we can only trust that whatever or however our baby is, we shall love him or her and be given the strength to live with whatever our lives deliver us. Yoga brings the strength of mind, body and emotions we need by developing what the Buddha called 'the natural mind': that which is behind and sustains the 'monkey mind' that runs all over the place, sometimes taking us with it. Ajahn Sucitto, at the Cittaviveka Buddhist Monastery (at Chithurst, in West Sussex, not far from where I live), correlates this natural mind with the core muscles that sustain the body, whereas the 'monkey mind' that meditation teachers speak of is likened to the outer muscles that move here and there.

There's a myriad of other concerns and worries that come up during this time, and they will be addressed throughout the book. There is much advice around, and yet yoga and meditation encourage us to look within, as all the knowledge we need for life is contained with our growing awareness at this time. In particular, we need to have faith in ourselves, and yoga enables this.

Maybe we also feel that society expects us to carry on as normal. In India and the rest of the 'East' they have a very different approach. They revere this time, and the woman carrying her precious cargo – a cargo that is growing and developing, becoming aware of its surroundings, and of the mother that is carrying the baby. The mother's awareness is also heightened to what is going on within her body and around her.

More than just help us make the right decisions, the practice of yoga in all its forms can enable us to develop just the awareness we need – or, to use the word associated with the Buddha, mindfulness. This means consciously feeling the enormous changes in the body and indeed in the whole self from the moment of conception, and going with those changes, listening within to what is needed. The changes will be different for each woman, as pregnancy (even each individual pregnancy) affects us in many different ways.

We can become very sensitive to our body and to the growing foetus within it and the soul that has come into us. One of the first memories I have is of feeling a sort of 'seal' come over the neck of the womb to contain the embryo. Of course I did not know I was pregnant at this stage, neither did I know, until much later, that this sealing actually happened physically: a plug does develop over the neck of the uterus (womb). This is an example of the greater increase in sensitivity to your body that accompanies pregnancy and subsequently motherhood.

Your baby is an evolved, sensitive being who is ready to be full of the purest love for you, the mother. If the essence of yoga is to be understood and practised, it is important to remember throughout your pregnancy the great privilege and honour of having been chosen to be a mother by the soul of your baby, and to tune in to the needs of the foetus inside you.

It is also helpful to remember that the soul coming to you has much to teach you. The bond between you as the mother and your child, created at this time, will always be there, even in miscarriage and death, and creates a firm foundation for the baby's time on earth, if that is to be.

So consciously communicate what you are doing and why you are doing it, and be awake to any response you feel from your baby, so that you intuitively know what is best for both of you. You will understand how it is possible to do this as you do it.

Another effect of pregnancy is to feel that our brains do not work as they have been used to working. This can be alarming, and I have realized from conversations with Sally that it is often talked about in midwifery. Pregnant women have been known to say, 'I have lost my brain', while midwives sometimes call it 'brain loss'. I feel this occurs partly because we are coming into our bodies more, and need to come into them, much more than our society based on the intellect generally allows us.

This can have advantages – one of my students with a very high-powered job in advertising found in pregnancy that all stress left her body and she totally relaxed as soon as she became pregnant. She could still do her job but her head didn't worry about it in the same way, as she was so centred in her body and what was happening to it.

I remember the great yoga teacher Sri BKS Iyengar saying that 'every cell of the body has intelligence if we use it'. The poor old head gets wound up in stress and worry, so take this as a wonderful opportunity to develop the intelligence and intuition of the body and heart. Pregnancy brings this, while yoga, mindfulness in daily life and meditation enhance, encourage and develop this awakening of heart and body.

WHO THIS BOOK IS FOR

This book is written for all those women who are interested in becoming pregnant, are trying to conceive, or are already pregnant, along with their loved ones and partners. It is also aimed at those in the midwifery profession who would like to offer yoga practice and advice for a happy, healthy pregnancy, and their colleagues in the public health nursing profession. This includes professionals connected to the National Childbirth Trust in the UK and its equivalents elsewhere, especially those who offer special classes and support to potential parents.

More than this, it is intended to support those parents, prospective parents and professionals who are interested in reducing the levels of intervention and painkillers in pregnancy, childbirth and postnatally – and in making it as natural and beautiful an event as possible.

Yoga gives us the ability to go with pain, thus reducing its power. It is often our resistance that intensifies pain and even creates it in the first place, whether the pain is physical, emotional or mental.

Much of the material that forms this book is taken from the pregnancy module in the courses run by the Inner Yoga Trust for yoga teachers who have already completed a general teacher training in yoga with the Trust, and it will be a handbook for that course. It is suitable, though, for all yoga teachers who want to give the best care to pregnant women through their teaching. It would also be helpful to anyone who is pregnant and wants to start or continue a practice of yoga, one that will enable them to have a relaxed, safe and enjoyable pregnancy with preparation for labour and for the postnatal time. In short, it's for all who have a personal or professional interest or a desire to help others in this wonderful event.

> *The most beautiful and most profound emotion we can experience is the*
> *sensation of the mystical. It is the sower of all true science.*
> Albert Einstein

USING THIS BOOK

It is advisable to have an experienced yoga teacher during pregnancy and after. Ideally this will be someone who has practised yoga herself during pregnancy and has done a pregnancy module in addition to a general teacher training.

Our society at the moment tends to encourage us to carry on as if nothing has changed – to continue maybe a heavy schedule of work, exercise, socializing and so on.

This is very different from the Indian system, which takes into account the enormous change in hormones – the increase in oestrogen and progesterone that takes place at the very beginning of pregnancy and then straight after giving birth a decrease in the oestrogen and progesterone, which means that much rest, awareness and gentleness are required at this time.

Yoga originates from India and developed the view that as well as matter (*prakriti* in Sanskrit) we are also energy (*purusha* in Sanskrit) thousands of years before modern physics started to hold it, through the brilliance of Albert Einstein and others who have followed in his direction. Science is gradually becoming familiar with the concept of energy that yoga holds, and is using it in all sorts of beneficial (and sometimes harmful) ways. In yoga philosophy the soul coming into this life is aware and strong in its energy body before it becomes aware in the physical body. Yet the practice of yoga helps us to develop precisely the awareness we need. We shall be following the Indian system in this book, and we will also encourage contact with the baby inside us through meditation, awareness and feeling the soul, spirit and consciousness of the baby.

DIAPHRAGMS

There are three main diaphragms in the body and they are all important in pregnancy. Their functions are to enable the breath to move in and out and to contain whatever is above them, and they are as follows.

1) The pelvic floor diaphragm
This a tendonous muscle that spreads across the floor of the pelvis from the pubic bone at the front to the coccyx (tailbone) at the back. It keeps the contents of the pelvis in place and works directly with the thoracic diaphragm (see diagram opposite) to create space in the abdomen, so that the breath then fills the chest cavity. As the thoracic diaphragm undulates out and down the pelvic diaphragm broadens and spreads. For the breath to go out these two diaphragms need to lift up into a dome,

to create less space so the breath has to be expelled.

2) The thoracic diaphragm
This attaches to the sides of the floating ribs and to the twelfth thoracic vertebra at the back and the bottom of the sternum (breastbone) at the front. Its

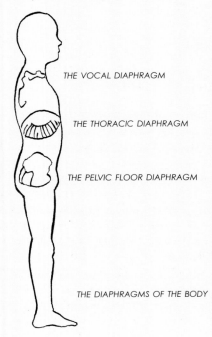

THE VOCAL DIAPHRAGM

THE THORACIC DIAPHRAGM

THE PELVIC FLOOR DIAPHRAGM

THE DIAPHRAGMS OF THE BODY

undulation, down and out, gives space for the lungs to fill with the breath. The following upward movement reduces the space in the chest cavity so that the air goes out.

It is a very strong tendonous muscle that also massages the heart as it moves.

3) The vocal diaphragm
This spreads across the vocal chords in the throat. It domes upwards with the inhalation to give more space for the lungs and relaxes with the exhalation, so enabling us speak or sing.

THE SUBTLE BODY

All ancient traditions teach awareness of more subtle bodies than the physical that interpenetrate the more solid physical body. We may have lost that awareness, but yoga practices will help us restore it. They will over time reconnect us with the subtle energy that runs through the body, which I mentioned earlier in this introduction. The whole concept of what is often referred to in western society as the

subtle body comes from the yoga system.

In Sanskrit, the language of the great texts of India such as the Vedas and the Upanishads, the bodies (whether physical or subtle) are referred to as kosas. A *kosa* is a veil of forgetting – of forgetting who we really are – translated as a 'sheath'.

A tiny baby forms first in what we may call its celestial body. In yoga the celestial body is the *ananda maya kosa* ('ananda' means bliss, and 'maya' means illusion). When you look into the eyes of a tiny baby – it feels as if they are all knowing, aware of all that you are and all that they are, and of the whole of existence.

The memory of having my daughter lying down beside me on the operating table a few minutes after she was born is still very much with me. She really looked deeply into my eyes – to see who it was who had been carrying her. I felt she knew me completely and knew 'what it was all about' – existence to be experienced. This lasts in a small baby for six months to a year, and it is stronger if the baby is breastfed, as it has then not taken nourishment from the earth, but feels instead quite heavenly.

When the baby is taking nourishment from the earth, it gradually becomes more solid, more 'of matter'. This is a coming into their more physical, solid, body, known in Sanskrit as *ana maya kosa*, in which 'ana' means food, so that they have literally become part of the earth, gradually losing their awareness of the *ananda maya kosa*, known not only as the celestial but also as the causal body, as it is the 'cause' of the other bodies. We get wrapped in day-to-day survival and what the ego wants in life, and forget what is the real purpose of living.

In between, the baby will have developed a subtle body that itself has three levels. One is the *vijnana maya kosa*, the body of knowledge. This is a blueprint for life, rather like DNA. Then there is the *mano maya kosa*, the mental body, which brings intelligence to every cell of the body. It is a recent discovery of neuroscience that every cell of the body has intelligence and awareness and can function as if it were the whole. The last of these three bodies is the *prana maya kosa*, the body of breath, *prana*. As we breathe, we can feel energy moving – this is a waking up of the subtle body connected with the breath, known as the *prana maya kosa*. The body of breath, or energy, is the one that we particularly become aware of through the practice of yoga.

The subtle bodies interpenetrate the physical body, and they give it life and awareness. As women we are all the more aware of these subtle bodies in pregnancy. As our awareness is then heightened to smells, noise and vibrations around us, we also become more conscious of what is happening within us. The subtle body wakes up as we take our attention to it!

There is a connection between the subtle body and the electrical impulses through the body that are sensitized in pregnancy. Electrical impulses create a magnetic field, and the magnetic field effectively forms the subtle body.

The practice of mindfulness yoga (yoga with awareness) channels this energy that runs through us, to balance and calm us, and to connect us to the growing foetus.

BANDHAS

The bandhas are at more or less the same level as the diaphragms, but they are more subtle in nature. In other words, they are part of the subtle body and movement of energy described on p. 16 under 'nadis'.

As we inhale, the whole body broadens and opens, and as we exhale there is a subtle doming up and arching out of the bandhas that lengthens the spine upwards from the base. The *mula bandha*, which is at the level of the pelvic floor, enables that direction of the spine and the energy in the spine to move upwards from the base, through the sacrum and into the lumbar spine. 'Mula' means base and 'bandha' means lock or containment, like a canal lock.

The *uddiyhana bandha* comes at the level of the thoracic diaphragm, and flies up and out to move the thoracic (upper) spine through the shoulderblades. The *jalandhara bandha*, at the level of the throat, lengthens the neck vertebrae up to support the head. Hence the whole body is transported and moved by the breath.

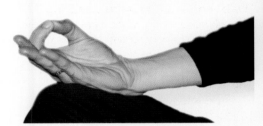

CHIN MUDRA: TIP OF THE THUMB
TO THE TIP OF THE INDEX FINGER

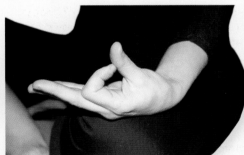

CHIN MUDRA: TIP OF THE INDEX
FINGER TO THE FIRST THUMB JOINT

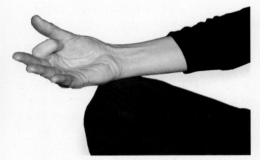

CHIN MUDRA: TIP OF THE INDEX FINGER
TO THE ROOT OF THE THUMB

MUDRAS

A mudra is a gesture or a stance. A *hasta mudra* is a gesture of the hand, where the fingers are held in such a way as to affect the energy running through the body. It creates a psycho-neural link back into the body, rather like the electrical connection made when you switch a light on. Here we are using a *hasta mudra* to connect to the diaphragms, to wake them up and so move them to encourage the breath to flow more easily and fully in and out.

The diaphragms and bandhas can be experienced and connected to by use

of the *chin mudra*. *Chin mudra* means a psychic gesture of consciousness.

In the first photo above Marielle has the tip of the index finger lightly touching the tip of the thumb, as she sits in the cross-legged meditation position, feeling the effect of the mudra. Traditionally it connects you to the pelvic floor diaphragm and the *mula bandha*, the one at the base of the spine, so the breath moves from there and brings awareness there.

In the second photo, she brings the index finger in to the first thumb joint nearest the nail. This traditionally connects your consciousness to the thoracic diaphragm and the *uddiyhana*

bandha, enhancing their action.

In the third position, the index finger is brought right in to the root of the thumb. This traditionally makes a connection with the vocal diaphragm and *jalandhara bandha,* the one in the throat.

A good starting point as you work with this book would be to use these mudras, and see what you feel. Don't worry if you feel none of the connections suggested, or feel something different. Trust your own awareness. It does, after all, take practice to develop such awareness, so we will be bringing the mudras in as you go through the practices set out in the book.

NADIS

These are energy channels in the body, and correspond to the meridians of Chinese medicine. We shall describe them as they arise in this the book, for instance on pp. 37–8, under the practice *Nadi sodhana*, which is a clearing and cleansing of the channels.

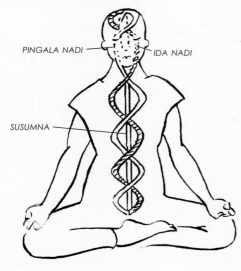

PINGALA NADI — IDA NADI

SUSUMNA —

THE NADIS

SOME SPECIAL TERMS

The front and back body
If we put a hand behind us we can feel the spinal processes at the back of the body. We therefore think that the spine is at the back. However the central axis of the spine runs right down the middle of the body, not at the back, and that part of the body which is behind or posterior to the axis of the spine is called the back body in yoga. The part which is in front of, or superior to, the central axis of the spine is termed the front body.

If the back body broadens and spreads in any posture, then the front body can relax and soften and open.

Spreading the sacrum
The sacrum consists of five fused vertebrae spread out to make a more solid bone with holes in it where the spaces would have been between the vertebrae. For a drawing of it see p. 104.

It joins onto the top of the pelvis, called the ilium, through the sacroiliac joint. This bone is said to fuse when you are around twenty-one years old. However it does spread during pregnancy, when the relaxin hormone is released. Then, the sacroiliac joint frees and opens to give space in the pelvis for the baby to move through.

So when in this book the instruction is to spread the sacrum, feel it opening out and back as though it slots into the pelvis better, for it tends to be held tight and contracted in.

You will find the word 'spread' used in a similar way in this book about the hands and feet and other parts of the body such as the shoulders. Use the same consciousness with this instruction: an awareness of spreading, opening, and aliveness.

THE INNER YOGA TRUST

The Inner Yoga Trust runs a three-year teacher's awareness programme. The course is structured as follows.

Year 1: A foundation course of seven weekends based on the structure of the textbook YOUR YOGA BODYMAP, sister volume to YOUR YOGA BIRTHGUIDE. This works from the feet up, connecting the feet to movements right through the body, with basic anatomy relative to movement and an outline of the wholeness of yoga as a life path.

Year 2: Here the focus is on one's own body and practice so that the teacher teaches from his or her own understanding. You do not need to want to teach in these two years; some students do these years in order to learn about themselves.

Year 3: In the third year, the focus moves to teaching from your own practice.

Years 2 and 3 both consist of five weekends and a week-long Summer School, all residential at various venues.

Courses are currently run by the School in the UK in Hampshire, Bristol, Kent, Surrey, Scotland, Ireland, Manchester, Shropshire and Cornwall.

The pregnancy module is taken after these three years if you want to run a pregnancy course or specialize in teaching pregnant women. It is being taught in Hampshire and Scotland at the present time. We are currently developing a children's module.

All courses are currently accredited by the British Wheel of Yoga, itself endorsed by Sport England.

PROFILES

This book has grown out of the courses offered by the Inner Yoga Trust, based at Petersfield, in Hampshire, England, and in particular its pregnancy module (see previous page). In this book we have throughout used student models from the school to illustrate the postures. Each pregnancy has its own story to tell, and although many students only appear in the book at one point in their pregnancy, others have been photographed at different stages, too. Here is a little more about the story of each.

 Paula McQueen is a paediatrician and thirty-seven years old. She gave birth to Bella on 28 December 2008 by caesarean section, so Bella was two and a half months old when the photos were taken. Paula has practised yoga for ten years.

 Her husband, Will Lane, at thirty-eight is a yoga teacher trained in the Inner Yoga School, a gardener and a Thai massage practitioner, and is seen with Bella too.

 Joy Hosie was six months pregnant and forty-four when the photos were taken. She gave birth to Amber (also in the photos) on 21 January 2009. She teaches yoga, has completed the Inner Yoga teachers' awareness programme and the pregnancy module, and is a tribunal judge in mental health and disability and a part-time musician.

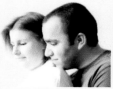 Kristy and John Perez-Vilas had Ellie on 25 May 2009. Kristy was seven months pregnant when the photos were taken. She is a sports therapist currently on the Inner Yoga teachers' awareness programme, and is thirty-three. John is a police officer, aged thirty-two.

 Panna Chittenden, forty-two, gave birth to Elliot by caesarean section on 9 May 2009, at the full moon in May which is the Buddha's birth, enlightment and death day. She was seven months pregnant when the photos were taken. Panna spent five years in Chithurst Buddhist Monastery as an Anagarika, preparing to be a nun. She has completed the Inner Yoga teachers' awareness programme, and has been a professional sailor as well as a climber and outdoor venturer. She is interested in rehabilitation through yoga after herself receiving head injuries from a bad cycling accident, and is currently training to be an occupational therapist.

Angela Ross was twenty-three weeks pregnant when photographed, her baby being due on 12 January 2010. Angela is thirty-three years old, works for a carers' charity, and has practised yoga for six years. She has just completed the Inner Yoga foundation course, and will go on to do the two-year teachers' awareness programme in Scotland, starting in March 2010 – on which her baby will accompany her.

 Tamsin Cowman has an English mother, Lyn Ng, who has taught yoga for many years, and a Chinese father, Michael Ng, an acupuncturist. Tamsin is thirty years old, and a Senior Nurse in Intensive Care at Frimley Park Hospital in Surrey, England. Zachary was born on 3 August 2009, so he was five and a half weeks old when the photos in the book were taken. Tamsin had to have a Caesarean section as she had a fibroid and her placenta would not detach, so her tummy has not yet returned to normal in her photos. Her yoga practice is expected to help this process. Her husband Chris (thirty-four) and son Samuel (three) practise yoga alongside Tamsin and appear in the photos.

 Karen, forty-two, was twelve weeks into her pregnancy when photos in the first trimester chapter were taken and eight months when she was photographed for the third trimester. Her baby is due in November 2009. She says that the practice of yoga has greatly supported her and given her trust in her own body.

 Saskia Snel is thirty-seven and gave birth to Sam on 28 August 2008, so her third trimester photos were taken at eight months, while Sam was nearly seven months when the postnatal photos taken. Saskia is a graphic designer and felt that yoga enabled her to have an easy and amazing, drug-free birth at home .

 Marielle Churaqui, forty-four, is an astrologer, reflexologist and yoga teacher specializing in pregnancy, postnatal yoga and mother and baby yoga. She is interested in conception and fertility issues.

 Emily Adsett, nineteen, was in her first trimester when the photos of her were taken. Her baby is due on 25 May 2010. She is an assistant teacher and has practised yoga for several years and will continue classes when she is fourteen weeks.

1. Conception

PREGNANCY is a time when our awareness of ourselves and the world around us, and maybe awareness of more subtle levels too, is naturally heightened. A heightening of awareness goes very well with the practice of yoga, as yoga works on the body and mind to wake them up to greater possibilities of life, movement, and sensitivity. Through our yoga practice we become more aware of what we really need to sustain and maintain our life, how our bodies need to move, how our energy is at the present, what we need to eat for vitality – all such important things in pregnancy.

If we already have a yoga practice, we might want to change it, perhaps drastically, especially in the first trimester (see the next chapter). It is important to be aware of how we feel, and that will tune us in to what is needed in our practice and in our lives.

Often, women who have never practised yoga before turn to yoga when pregnant rather than to other forms of exercise. Many make this choice to prepare for the birth, as the movement and suppleness yoga brings can help tremendously in labour and childbirth. It also helps the mind go with the whole process through difficulties and pain (see chapter 5, on Labour). We need to be able to listen to what we naturally need and so come out of driving and pushing ourselves hard at this time. Instead we need to learn to relax. Yoga enables this.

THE TIME OF CONCEPTION

The time around conception can be a sensitive one, especially when a baby is very much wanted. We can become very aware and open to what is happening in our bodies, and maybe in our partners' too, but also around us, as energies come together for this momentous occasion. We may be aware at the time of an immediate change – even of the sperm entering the egg – and then afterwards as every part of our body shifts to accommodate this change.

Yoga can be of great assistance at the time of conception. First, it allows us time to relax by providing postures, breathing and meditation that enable and enhance this, and secondly it can make us more conscious beings.

Of course, it is all very well to say 'sit down and relax' to someone, and even to yourself; but if we have been overcharged and have a very busy life, relaxation often does not come that easily. It is often easier to find relaxation in the postures than simply 'relaxing', or by adopting the relaxation pose.

My own observation as a yoga teacher is that in women who are having difficulty conceiving, the whole lower abdomen is often in some way contracted or 'held'; to put it another way, it is as if there is no vitality there. There can be many reasons for this, both psychological and physical. For example, high-heeled shoes and tight jeans push the pelvis forward and constrict the ovaries. The yoga postures can gently work to release the causes of any blocks at both the physical and energetic levels, and there will be a consequent benefit at all levels, a benefit which will come subtly and gently.

There may be other, linked medical problems. For instance, diverticulitis is a condition of the bowel that can have an affect on the whole of this area of the body. I have known students with diverticulitis whom regular yoga practice has helped, and who have then gone on to conceive, long after they began trying.

Some suggest that the contraceptive pill, taken over long periods, can affect successful conception. Homeopathy is said to help this, but yoga postures too will help to clear the effects.

As for men, who don't get a lot of attention in this book, for obvious reasons, their blood supply to the testes and prostate area can be increased by practising the postures in a way that relaxes the pelvis back (which is how they are taught in this book). This in turn can improve the sperm count.

Any form of abuse can affect both women and men adversely – at physical, psychological and energetic levels. Again, yoga can work on the physical and subtle bodies to release these memories. Through yoga, they are held and soothed in a gentle way, gradually dissolving them and usually without the need to analyse any memories that can surface through yoga.

EXPLORING

If there is difficulty conceiving (see p. 25), we need as teachers to explore with students other avenues beside yoga, although many of them connect back to it.

Just as yoga explores the energy lines of the body (in Sanskrit, they are called *nadis* – see p. 15), I have myself been helped by exploring the energy lines of the earth. Thus, I might visit a sacred site such as a stone circle where you can walk and sit among the stones. One friend told me how a trip to Callanish, a stone circle on Lewis, one of the islands of the Outer Hebrides in Scotland, helped her, while another talked about how she had gone to Cairnpaple and the Clinking Stanes near Edinburgh. Round about the time I conceived, I actually went through the fertility stone Men-an-Tol in the west of Cornwall (shown below). Our understanding of how this might be, how people are helped to conceive by these visits, is very limited; but who can tell what knowledge people who built circles of quite extraordinary astronomical complexity may have had around the matter of fertility?

There is a connection at many of these stone circles to the movement of the moon as well as to the sun. Recent research at both Stonehenge and Callanish has shown accurate and detailed positioning of the stones on the site (and in the surrounding area at Callanish, and in the long barrows around Stonehenge), to make them line up with the extreme positions of the moon over its eighteen-year cycle. The monthly cycle of a woman has also been linked to the moon as it is the same length as the moon's progress from new to full and back to new again.

Astrologers say that a woman would naturally menstruate in line with the phase the moon had reached when she was born. It has been shown that when women are in a group situation such as a nunnery, they tend to adapt their time of menstruation to the extent that they menstruate more or less together, that is, at the

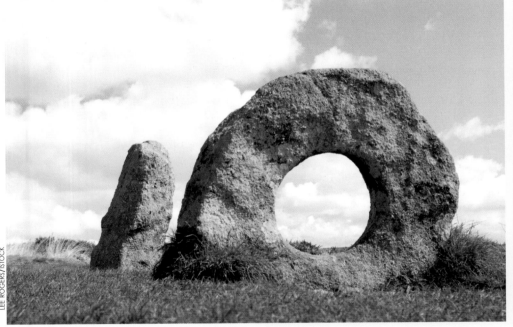

LEE ROGERS/ISTOCK

same actual phase of the moon, not the time dictated by their birth rhythm.

Maybe there is a link here to the natural rhythm of a woman's cycle and to the times that she is most likely to conceive. Equipment can now be bought in the local chemist to measure the most likely time for a woman to conceive. Maybe a ritual can be developed at this time of noting the phase of the moon and meditating with it, inside or outside in some open high place where the moon is vis-

ible. We can then become aware of how the phases of the moon can affect us.

LATER IN LIFE

Both men and women are often healthier and fitter today because of the better diet and exercise levels that arise from higher standards of living, so that having a family later in life is more possible than it once was. There is an increasing trend to

leave having children until a career and certain level of lifestyle and even more, maybe, till a greater sense of self has been established. Yet there is also concern today that sedentary lifestyles render other mothers so unfit that it is actually becoming more difficult for them to carry a baby comfortably and to give birth.

I was almost forty-one when my own child, Beth, was born. It has been said to me that older parents are more patient and have more wisdom, while younger ones are fitter and have more energy to deal with their babies and young children. Older parents can be an embarrassment to teenagers, as my own daughter found, but then to anyone in their teens all parents are generally an embarrassment!

All in all, despite the risks the medical profession rightly notes, it may be just as well to wait if you wish. In fact, a baby will come when he or she knows at a deep level that the time is right for all, though with our busy minds we may not be able to be so aware of that moment. From a spiritual viewpoint, the outcome of the greater inherent risks – such as a Down's syndrome baby – may

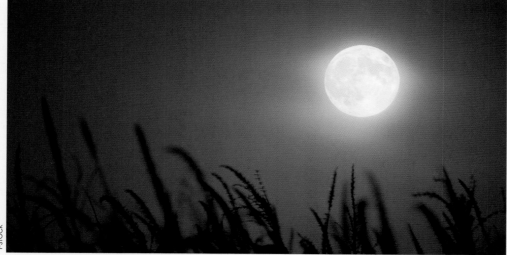

I-STOCK

actually be what is needed, karmically, although I recognize that I am making a very controversial statement here. We cannot know, though, what unexpected blessings apparent misfortunes may bring. Because of the higher statistical likelihood of abnormality associated with late conceiving, we need great care about conceiving and awareness of whether we would be willing to have such a special child and whether we feel we could give them the appropriate upbringing and home.

I was aware of my own biological clock running out when I turned forty, and that subconsciously influenced me, or so I felt in hindsight. I had read a Chinese book that stated 'an older woman, if she wants to conceive, needs to choose a younger man – then she will have a healthy, intelligent child'. In China they apparently call it 'a May–September relationship'. I felt the influence of this statement, though not very consciously until I was pregnant – and yet I had been told that I would be unable to conceive. That influenced me, too!

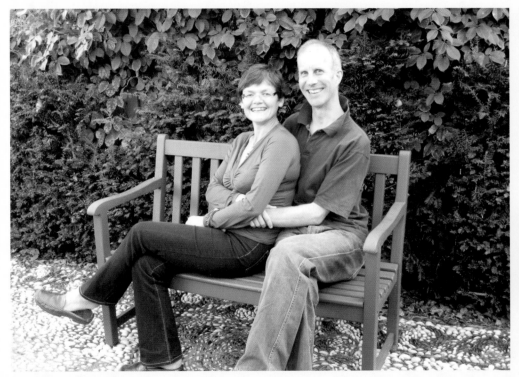

DIFFICULTIES WITH CONCEIVING

No-one is entirely sure of the reason some women have difficulty conceiving, if no specific medical problem has been diagnosed. Yoga has been thought to help for the reason that certain postures can increase blood supply to the ovaries.

Many women now choose to start a family later in life – beyond the age of thirty – when a reason for not conceiving is often that the eggs are older and less mobile. The main cause of this is stress, and women need active encouragement to relax and allow pregnancy to happen, free of guilt and other social pressures.

It's important that while yoga may help when there are difficulties in conceiving, doing yoga postures must not be seen as a 'cure'; proper advice should be sought, and the postures practised alongside any medical recommendations.

FEARS

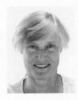

For many, pregnancy brings on enormous fears, such as 'will my child be normal?'. What follows are some words written by one of the Inner Yoga Trust's teachers about his Down's syndrome child, but there is more about what we perhaps wrongly call abnormality in the postnatal chapter, on p. 121.

'The combination of Simone's age

and the nuchal fold measurement, taken at the twelve-week scan, gave a probability of one in fifteen that our second child had Down's syndrome. The hospital staff clearly expected us to want a more conclusive test, with a view to aborting the child should that prove positive; not a route we wished to take. Fearing the truth, perhaps, I talked myself into believing that the child would be "normal". That Jaru did indeed have Down's syndrome, came as a rude shock despite the warning.

'Has yoga helped in coming to terms with his condition? Undoubtedly, without my asana practice I would have been even more inflexible, in both body and mind, less able to adapt. Also, at the times that I have been more consistent in some form of meditative practice, I believe that I have been better able to take potential stressors in my stride.

'Ultimately, though, the greatest help has been Jaru himself. His radiant presence is an absolute delight. Certainly, we have been very fortunate that he has avoided the most serious of the health problems associated with the condition. Above all, what he is teaching

us, though, is that the most painful part of having a child with Down's syndrome is not the reality but our presumptions and preconceptions, and our tendency to cling to those despite the reality. Before Jaru's birth, whenever I had seen someone with Down's syndrome, I saw the syndrome, not the individual. Now I am beginning to meet individuals, one of whom I am proud to say is my son.'

CONCEPTION-PHASE POSTURES

The next few pages contain a selection of postures that further the opening of the blood supply to the ovaries in women and the testes in men, and to the lower abdominal area generally, and so may help in conception.

All the postures given for the conception phase will be of benefit for men, too. This is true of all the postures of yoga, so long as the pelvis is relaxed and spread back, as described in the Introduction, p. 16. We often tilt the pelvis forward, but it needs to be in line with the ankles and knees. For a fuller discussion of this, see my earlier book, YOUR YOGA BODYMAP FOR VITALITY.

I. VIRASANA AND SUPTA VIRASANA
SITTING HERO AND HERO-TO-LYING-BACK POSE

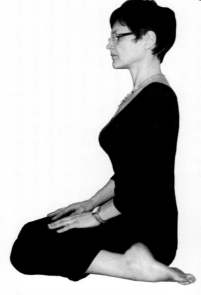

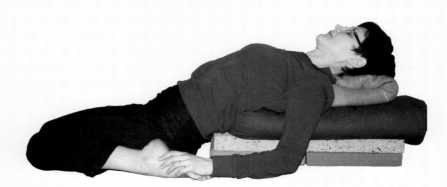

These postures can be practised to open out the lower abdominal area. You will need a range of supports behind you to go back onto.

Sit down on the knees as Marielle is doing in the lefthand photograph below. If there is any strain on your knees, hips or feet, put a block under your buttocks. Lengthen the spine out of the hips.

Feel the spread this gives across the abdominal area.

Lift up and forward through the upper back to give a gentle back bend. Spread the back body back onto the support as in the second photograph, so that there is no strain on the back or neck.

In the photograph on the next page, Marielle is having her pelvis gently relaxed back to release the lumbar spine and lower abdomen. Pressure from the hands of your partner or teacher can be very helpful for the hips and this whole area.

Relax in the lying-back position for as long as is comfortable – it can be for up to fifteen minutes.

When you are ready to move, take your hands firmly down beside you and lift the whole upper body to come up and go forward into the next posture.

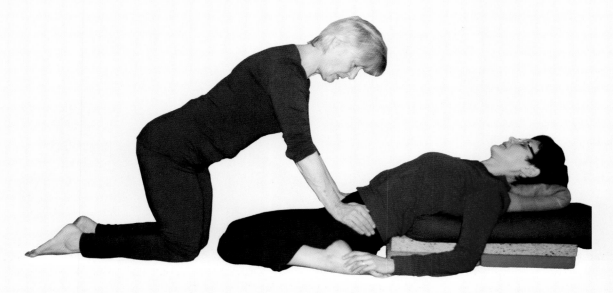

2. PINDASANA
CHILD OR EMBRYO POSE

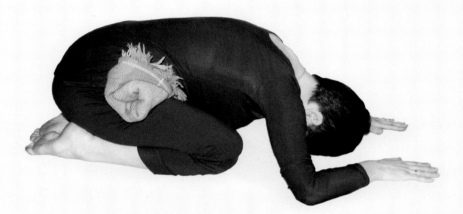

Kneeling on the ground, roll the coccyx (tailbone) back over the heels and then rest the spine forward and down so that the crown of your head comes to the ground. You will find that resting your head on the earth relaxes the mind. Again, stay as long as is comfortable: it could be fifteen minutes if you are tired or suffer from insomnia. As you rest into the pose and gently breathe, feel the spread of the diaphragms across the pelvic floor and across the lower ribs, so that your breathing comes from the movement of your diaphragms. This greatly increases the circulation of the blood around your whole system as the thoracic diaphragm is connected to the heart and helps it pump blood around the body. Spread down through your feet and legs and back into your sacrum to bring the whole spine up as one, and then stretch your legs forward to go into the next pose.

It can be helpful to have a rolled blanket placed across the top of your thighs, to spread the belly more as shown in the photo.

3. Upavistha Konasana
WIDE ANGLE POSE

From the previous pose, take the legs wide, as Marielle is doing. Stretch one arm up and out of the hip and overhead to lift the hip, and then relax it down to make more space around the sacrum and abdominal area. Then, relaxing forward and keeping the spine straight and knees relaxed, breathe gently from the diaphragms so that you feel the back ribs opening away from the spine, which allows the spine to lengthen forward and up.

There are some variations on this posture on p. 154.

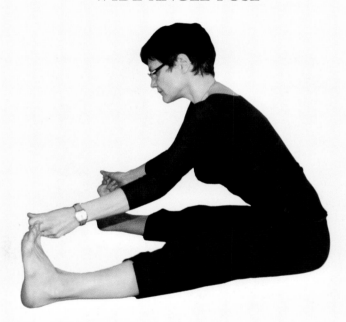

Points to watch: *lengthen back from the heels into the hips to bring the head of the femur deep into the hip socket. This brings the* mula bandha *and base diaphragm naturally in, to free the abdominal area and lengthen the spine up. Keep the spine lengthened and the shoulders relaxed down, also to open out the abdominal area.*

4. BADDHA KONASANA FROM UPAVISTHA KONASANA
CAUGHT ANGLE OR COBBLER POSE

Bring the soles of your feet together as shown. Lengthen your spine and rest there, feeling the opening in your hips and sacrum.

Then, extending forward from the base of the spine, as in the second photo, spread your hands down so that the spine lengthens forward and up through the shoulders.

When you are ready to come out of the pose spread back into the sacrum to come upright and take your hands around the outside of your knees to bring them together.

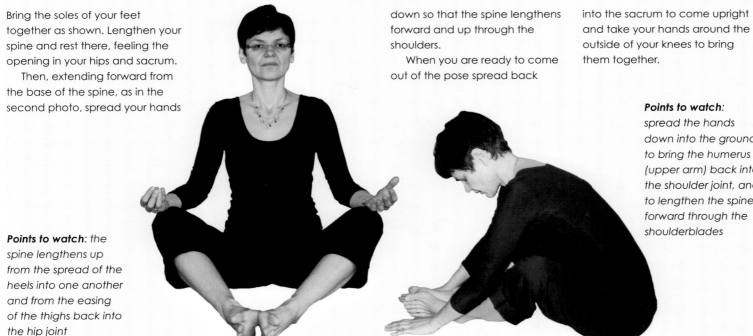

Points to watch: *the spine lengthens up from the spread of the heels into one another and from the easing of the thighs back into the hip joint*

Points to watch: *spread the hands down into the ground to bring the humerus (upper arm) back into the shoulder joint, and to lengthen the spine forward through the shoulderblades*

5. Janu Sirsasana
HEAD TO KNEE POSE

Points to watch: *keep the heels spreading to lengthen spine and tummy*

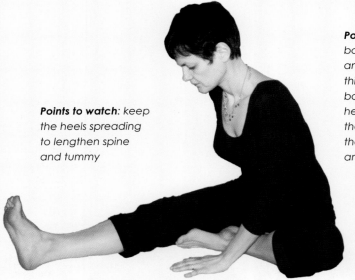

Points to watch: *have both heels extending and working. The thighbone easing back into the hip joint helps the turn over the straight leg. Keep the spine forward and up*

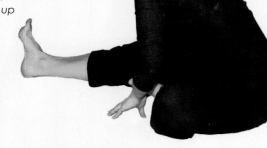

Janu sirsasana translates as head to knee pose, but it is much better on the spine if the spine is lengthened forward and up rather than down.

From *Baddha Konasana*, lengthen out one leg and let the other leg bend out to the side as shown. Now twist from deep in the sacrum up to the kidney, first towards the bent leg and then towards the straight leg. Then go forward over the straight leg, keeping space in the abdominal area and the spine lengthened forward and up.

Repeat on the other side.

If the lower spine rolls back or the straight leg is under strain, put some support under the knee as shown in the next pose, or bend the knee with the foot on the ground.

6. PASCHIMOTTANASANA
SITTING FORWARD BEND

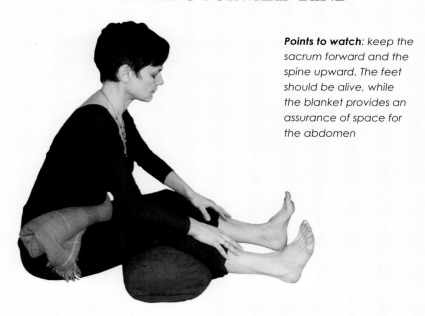

Points to watch*: keep the sacrum forward and the spine upward. The feet should be alive, while the blanket provides an assurance of space for the abdomen*

Still sitting on the mat, lengthen out both legs to *Dandasana*, Staff pose (see p. 90). Take the whole spine forward from the base, keeping the abdomen area soft with the support of a blanket across the tops of legs to lift over and thus give space across the abdomen, as in the photograph. If the kneecap pushes back into the leg this will make the back curve, so also put a bolster or rolled blanket under the legs as shown. To come back to *Dandasana* bring the whole spine up and back as one.

7. Setu Bandha Sarvangasana
BRIDGE POSE

Points to watch: keep the abdomen relaxed back and spreading and the throat relaxed and open. The shoulders drop down and the spine moves towards the head

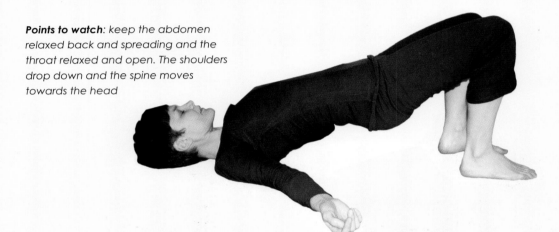

From *Paschimottanasana*, lie down on your back with knees bent and feet flat on ground. Spread down into your feet, especially the heels, lifting up through the shin bones, so that your pelvis lifts. This comes from using the legs and feet so that the lower back does not push at all. Then move the whole spine forwards towards the head.

It is good to go in and out of this pose several times, as each time you will come up more from your feet and legs and the whole pelvis area can rest down like a hammock, so that there is a movement away of the knees and forward of the spine towards the head, rather than pushing the pelvis up, which we tend to do to try and get there.

Rest your back down in between each repeat of the posture and before moving onto the next, so that you can feel the life in your spine and the resting and softening of the abdomen.

8. Salamba Sarvangasana
SHOULDERSTAND

Points to watch: *keep the feet active, the hips over the shoulders, and the arms spreading down and away to lift the back*

Points to watch: *spread up and into the heels to work legs, and so to lift up*

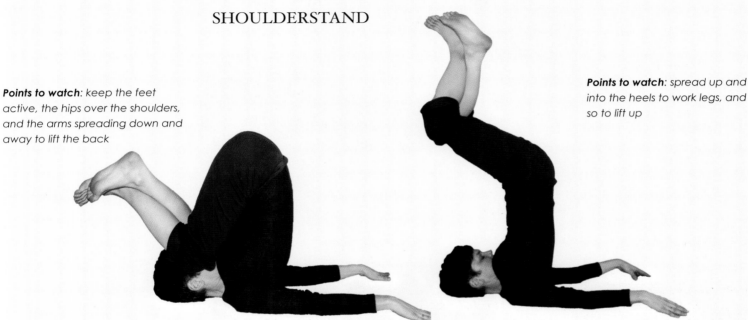

For *Salamba sarvangasana* (Shoulderstand), either bring your legs up and over your head or, if you need a little more momentum, come back to *Paschimottanasana* and roll back and over so that your legs are crossed over your face, as shown. This will relax the abdomen.

Now, using the cross of the legs gradually to stretch up as shown, move into Shoulderstand with the legs lifting you up. Stay there as long as the legs are lifting you so that there is no heaviness on your neck. Spread the upper arms down to help the lift.

When you are ready to come down, spread the arms and hands firmly into the ground, so that the back comes down gradually.

9. SAVASANA AND NADI SODHANA
RELAXATION AND ALTERNATE NOSTRIL BREATHING

From Shoulderstand, lie back down with a blanket under your knees to relax back down, and a block under each heel as shown, as this enables the whole belly area to relax back. You may also need a lift under the head if your neck is under strain and your head drops back. Let your whole body rest back and be supported by the ground so the front body rests

back into the back body.

Nadi sodhana literally means cleansing of the energy channels in the body but is also called alternate nostril breathing. Lie in *Savasana* with your hands on the lower abdomen as shown. As you lift the left hand (inset picture) feel the breath is encouraged into the left side of the body, the left lung and left nostril, then let it go out

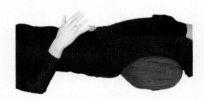

through the right side. Rest the left hand down and lift the right hand to encourage the breath in the right side, and exhale through the

left side. Repeat this as many times as it feels your awareness can stay with it. Then breathe easily through both nostrils, feeling the greater expansion of the breath through the body.

When you are ready to come up, roll onto one side, rest there a moment, and then come up from your side to sitting.

Points to watch: *the shoulders are relaxed down. A bolster under the knee relaxes the pelvis back so that the abdomen has space*

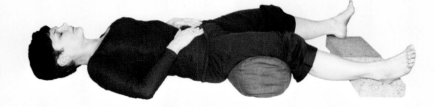

10. NADI SODHANA, SITTING
CLEANSING OF THE ENERGY CHANNELS

When you feel at ease and aware of the practice of *Nadi sodhana* lying down, you may like to do it sitting. Sit in any comfortable posture: in the photo, Marielle is in the seated mountain cross-legged posture and using the lotus mudra shown (for more on mudras see pp. 15 and 38). To do this, close all the fingers in, to touch the thumb, using lotus mudra (shown in detail at right).

As your breath comes in, open the fingers of your left hand and feel if the breath is more emphasized through the left nostril into the left lung. Gently exhale, again feeling the left nostril. Repeat for a few more breaths on this side, and then do a few breaths on the right side.

Now, opening the fingers of the left hand, breathe in to the top of

the inhalation without straining, closing the fingers on the left as you do so. Open the fingers of the right hand and exhale through the right side. Inhale through the right side, and at the top of the inhalation close the fingers on the right. Open them on the left as you exhale through the left side.

Do not hold your breath, so make the

Points to watch: *keep the feet active to support legs and back. The spine lengthens up from the life in the legs and feet*

change of position of the fingers gradually throughout each breath. Repeat the sequence as many times as feels comfortable without straining. Return to breathing gently through both nostrils, feeling as you do so whether the nostrils have cleared.

Lie down again after you finish and rest for a few

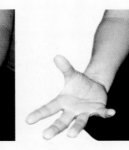

minutes; you could then move on to meditation (see overleaf).

The nadis are the channels of energy that move through the body, and this breathing clears those channels so that both the breath and the energy (*prana* in Sanskrit) move easily through the body after this practice.

This breath will work to clear the head and the endocrine glands, and especially the pituitary gland, situated deep in the skull – the gland which links to conception.

11. Meditation
with Mudra

Sit in a comfortable asana for you – that is, either cross the legs or kneel, or sit on a chair if the other postures are not easy to stay in for ten to thirty minutes.

Marielle's hands are shown here in *shakti mudra*. Mudras, which we met first on p. 16, relate to the gestures or stances that we might habitually find ourselves in as a result of our *samskaras*, those habitual waves of thought that build up day by day and (to continue the metaphor) create sandbanks in the mind and body, that become our conditioning and our everyday habits. These can be habits of bodily posture or the way we place our hands, and they say a lot about who we are, how we are and what impression we want to give to others.

A habitually strained posture would eventually create a strain or lack of ease in the body that would lead to the body not functioning as it should do and to dis-ease. Changing the posture would release the strain and heal the body. However, habits that have been with us a long time are not always easy to break. This may be gradually achieved through the postures of yoga and through our moment-by-moment awareness of the body and how we are standing, sitting, walking.

Mudras and especially *hasta mudras* (hand mudras) can greatly increase the effect of yoga in all its aspects. Just as the feet have all the nerve endings and energy channels running through them (which is what many therapies use), so do the hands.

This rather intricate *shakti mudra*

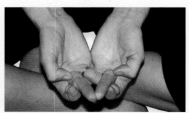

stimulates the feminine energy that resides in the base and sacral area at the level of the reproductive organs. Shakti is the goddess of fertility in the Vedic scriptures; a place sacred to her, under her name of Parvati, is shown in the photo opposite.

Bring the middle fingers together, so that the fourth and fifth finger link, then loop the index around the opposite fourth finger, bringing the tip of the thumb to the root of the middle finger, as shown. Rest the hands in your lap, as though they were a chalice.

Bring your awareness to your breath moving through your body. Don't interfere with it: let it find its way in then gently go out. Let the mind ride on the wave of the breath until there is a settling feeling in mind, body and emotions.

Feel the effect of the mudra on your breath and on your mind and awareness. Is there a sense of a circuit of energy from the base of the spine up through the left side of the body and across the brow, then down through the right side of the body, back to the base of the spine? Stay with this feeling for as long as you feel able to, bringing the mind back when it goes off on a topic. The time may be short at first and then increase and vary a lot from day to day. If it becomes a regular practice, it will have a gradually increasing effect of understanding and acceptance on mind, body and spirit.

We cannot say that the practice given here will enable you to conceive. However, I have known people who have conceived and others who have not who nonetheless have been greatly helped. It will certainly bring support, understanding and acceptance to your whole life.

It would be very helpful to have a teacher who could instruct you in this practice, as there are many subtle movements of the body that make such a difference to the energy and so the whole system. Since the practice is individual to each person, not everything can be put into writing: it takes a skilled teacher to see the uniqueness of the student. Do get in touch with the Inner Yoga Trust if you would like to find an IYT teacher in your area to help you develop this practice.

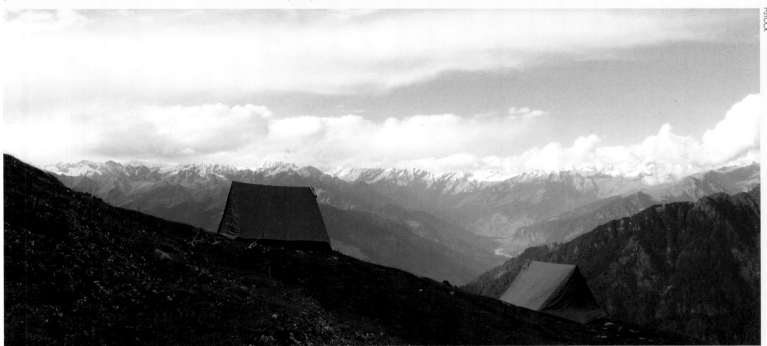

I-STOCK

IVF
IN VITRO FERTILIZATION

The sequence just described would help an IVF programme at the ovarian stimulation and egg retrieval phase, up to the point of the egg being implanted back into the womb.

An IVF programme can be very stressful as it would follow a long period of not conceiving, and the decision to embark on this programme is a great expense of finances and time. There are often discouraging opinions given by others, so we need to be strong in our own convictions here. Again, yoga practice encourages this. Moreover, a large quantity of hormones are injected to bring on menopause to the natural system so that the IVF programme can take over. The practices of yoga in all their aspects – philosophical, physical

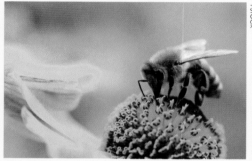

I-STOCK

MANKIND IS THE HONEY OF ALL BEINGS; ALL BEINGS THE HONEY OF MANKIND.
THE BRIGHT ETERNAL SELF THAT IS IN MANKIND,
THE BRIGHT ETERNAL SELF THAT LIVES IN A MAN OR A WOMAN, ARE ONE AND THE SAME; THAT IS IMMORTALITY, THAT IS SPIRIT, THAT IS ALL.
BRIHADARANYAKA UPANISHAD
('FAMOUS DEBATES IN THE FOREST')
TRANS. SRI PUROHIT SWAMI AND WB YEATS

and mental – can help enormously to aid the success of this programme.

Great care needs to be taken after the implant of the egg. Relaxation, breathing and meditation, in the ways set out in the next chapter (on the first trimester) are best at this time. It would be better to work with a skilled, experienced yoga teacher; please contact the Inner Yoga Trust if you would like to find one in your area.

A helpful meditation would be to sit with awareness of your breath moving through your body, particularly focusing on the thoracic diaphragm moving and back ribs spreading away from the spine, and then to visualize life, awareness, light in the form of a flame, in the uterus area.

MISCARRIAGE

Unfortunately, fifteen percent of all pregnancies end in miscarriage, which is defined as 'the involuntary loss of the products of conception prior to twenty-four weeks' gestation'. There are a variety of reasons for miscarriage, which include foetal abnormality (if determined), maternal age, infection, maternal disease and environmental factors. Some we can help with and some we cannot. Whether as midwives or as yoga teachers, the most we can do is give empathetic support and possibly recommend counselling.

My colleague Janis Binnie describes the agony she went through following the miscarriage of her first child.

'I know from personal experience that there is overwhelming grief. I remember in the

THERE WAS NEVER A TIME WHEN I DID NOT EXIST, NOR YOU, NOR ANY BEING. NOR IS THERE ANY FUTURE IN WHICH WE SHALL CEASE TO BE. THAT WHICH IS NON-EXISTENT CAN NEVER COME INTO BEING, THAT WHICH IS CAN NEVER CEASE TO BE. THAT REALITY WHICH PERVADES THE UNIVERSE IS INDESTRUCTIBLE. NO ONE HAS THE POWER TO CHANGE THE CHANGELESS.
BHAGAVAD GITA
(FROM SRI KRISHNA, THE YOGA OF KNOWLEDGE)

The Bhagavad Gita, first written down over 2500 years ago, is completely in line with modern physics, which states that energy cannot be destroyed or made, only transferred. Hence Albert Einstein's famous equation, $e=mc^2$, where e is energy, m is matter, and c is the speed of light.

first few weeks how unbearably physical the loss felt – I have never felt more like a wounded animal than I did in the weeks immediately following my miscarriage. The foetal position was ever a refuge.

As were the silent tears. The first few periods were physically and emotionally debilitating. I remember how very few people could acknowledge my loss, how few were able to even touch on the grief and emptiness I felt. Two weeks after my miscarriage my sister-in-law, bless her, found me crying in my mother's kitchen on Christmas Day trying to escape from the family world of congenial happiness, and blithely quipped "never mind, you'll soon be pregnant again".

'So many women experience miscarriage, at least once. I understand, from all the books I read at the time, that fifty percent of all first pregnancies end in miscarriage. I don't how many of these miscarriages are in the first six weeks of a pregnancy when, perhaps, the loss is less pronounced than when a pregnancy has progressed further.

'Despite this high incidence, women are simply advised to pick themselves up, to get over it as quickly as possible and look forward to being pregnant again.'

If you miscarry, or a student or client miscarries, it is like a physical death of a precious baby that has been growing inside you – and yet, at the same time, your body is going through the motions of still being pregnant. So the body needs to go though that process of pregnancy while the mind and soul deal with the grief of loss. Very gentle yoga postures can help here, those shown for conception as well as those shown for pregnancy, especially those supported restorative postures shown with bolsters and support to let the body recover and the mind adjust and somehow understand why the soul came so near and yet not right to you. My colleague Pauline says;.

'Miscarriage at whatever stage it happens is a traumatic experience (not only for us but for those around us – family and friends) and having personally been through three at varying stages I always had a strong sense of their spirit (and still occasionally do). On my last pregnancy, which went to just over seven months, I had a strong sense of my baby that

that was all he needed: just this brief experience in incarnation. Of course there are many reasons why miscarriages happen, many causes of miscarriage, but I found this concept helpful: that the incoming soul may be just needing one brief experience of incarnation. In all three cases I was aware of the importance of naming the babies I had 'lost', something which helped during my grief and sense of loss.

'With regard to the body, as Jenny teaches, great care needs to be taken. The length of time spent in rest and nurturing will be determined by the stage at which the miscarriage happened. Hormones, ligaments and oestrogen levels all need to find again their normal state. Relating emotionally and intimately needs gentle careful handling. Emotions such as anger, shame and guilt, to name just a few, are likely to arise.

'Meditation, visualization and eventually a gentle yoga practice help enormously in the healing process, bringing an inner strength and acceptance.'

Having read the profound words from

the Bhagavad Gita overleaf, sit with your feelings about this sad event. Have the courage to let them surface. Let tears flow if they come, let anger be there if it needs to be, as though you could hold all those myriad feelings in the palm of your hand. When those feelings begin to subside, see the soul that came close to you but not right into this life. This may be as a light, a bird that does not touch the earth or as a tiny baby. Know that that soul knows you, and for some reason has made contact with you, come close to you. What is it for you to experience and understand here, to take with you on your life's journey?

There have been many recorded experiences of women or others around them being able to feel or even see a soul with those who have miscarried. Trust these feelings, however unlikely they may seem in our rational, concrete world. Finish your meditation by giving thanks for that experience, even though very painful. There is a blessing for you there, and you can be enriched by that experience when you let go of bitterness, envy and resentment and feel the preciousness of it.

TERMINATION

There are going to be times when it does not feel appropriate to bring a baby into our current circumstances, maybe because we are unable to give a home, or what we would think of as a good home, to a baby, or because we do not have the love and support needed. Whatever the reason, it is the choice of the woman carrying the baby to act in her own best interests and that of the foetus.

Once again, the practice of yoga before and after termination can bring more acceptance of the situation as it is. Santosa is one of the Eight Limbs of Yoga, and it means acceptance or contentment. Yoga practice, especially breathing and meditation, can take

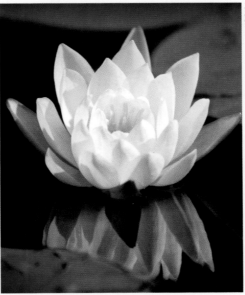

THE LOTUS LEAF RESTS UNWETTED ON WATER
BHAGAVAD GITA
(FROM SRI KRISHNA, THE YOGA OF RENUNCIATION)

us through the after-effects of the operation.

Guilt and regret about a termination can stay with one for a time – sometimes for life – and can surface when a pregnancy that is more appropriate in its timing comes along. So there is a need to work with these feelings of regret and guilt by sitting and letting them surface and honestly acknowledging them and feeling what comes out of them.

Once the feelings have been allowed to be, breathe with them and feel your diaphragm and solar plexus area open and release and move with your breath. Often it is in this area that feelings are held. Perhaps some purpose or sense will come from this quiet sitting as a result of that earlier event.

To Do the Postures or Not to Do the Postures

Some yoga schools such as the Iyengar one recommend that you do no yoga postures at all in the first trimester, which we come to next. This is because it is the time when miscarriage is most likely to happen. Whether you are a pregnant woman, a yoga teacher or a midwife, you may feel you want to go with this tradition and not do any postures, or teach them, until after fourteen weeks (twelve to fourteen weeks being the most common time for miscarriage).

If you have, or the one in your care has, a history of miscarriage I would recommend sticking to this basic rule. However, more recent research has shown that miscarriage comes from within the system of mother and baby, not outside it, so perhaps as yoga teachers we do not need to have the fear around it we may have been taught to feel?

It is also a standard recommendation that if you have practised yoga before you became pregnant, then you can carry on doing whatever your practice was before the pregnancy began, in the first trimester, so long as your body feels comfortable doing it. Often women who do other forms of exercise before they became pregnant will turn to yoga at this time as it is very helpful to labour. It needs stressing that it's not always the easy option! So care is needed. Yoga is so different from other forms of movement, as it works inwardly on the core of the body and with the energy of the body.

As women, we also need to be really guided by our inner voice. Outer authorities can be rather masculine for us, particularly at this time of sensitivity. Our inner voice – our awareness or intuition, so long as we can hear it – knows exactly what is best for us as individuals, and this might be quite different from what is right for the next woman. This is especially evident when women are pregnant as the responses in their bodies to that change are so diverse. Some women need *not* to do the postures; some can do whatever their body feels like. In the main, though, there will be distinct exceptions. I have often found that inverted postures, for instance, especially Dog pose and parts of Salutation to the Sun, can make the face flushed in this period. Never do a pose that feels wrong to you or which produces that flushing.

We also need to bear in mind that some women may not know they are pregnant until ten weeks and others may prefer to keep it to themselves until after fourteen weeks, so yoga teachers need always to keep aware in a class to note any changes. Noting these changes is part of yoga teaching anyway, but very important around pregnancy and childbirth. Often you can tell intuitively or by subtle changes in bearing so be aware and trust your 'tuition from within', the intuition.

2. The First Trimester: One to Three Months

HOW WOMEN feel during the first phase of their pregnancy varies enormously. Some feel so tired that they just want to lie down for the three months, others don't feel any symptoms. Some have morning sickness or even all-day sickness. So it is very important to listen to your body and follow what it seems to need.

Pregnancy in any circumstances can come as something of a shock! My own response was utter surprise. I was teaching yoga and taking part in a relationships course on the island of Hawaii. It took me quite a while to adapt to the news and I felt quite ill at first – owing more to shock and fear, I think, than bodily changes – yet at the same time it felt somehow very special, precious and important. Once I had adapted I was very excited and buoyed up by what was happening to my body and the awareness of this precious life inside it. It can be worth remembering that even in a wanted pregnancy (and often an initially unwanted pregnancy can in a short time become very wanted), there is still a moment when it all seems unbelievable and impossible. This is not surprising, as the change it creates in your life is monumental and forever. So time is needed to adjust; to accommodate this new state and go with it.

A rebalancing of lifestyle is important in early pregnancy. The rapidly growing foetus develops all its major organs in the first twelve weeks, so environmental factors are particularly important at this stage. Advice on diet is outside the scope of this book, but this, and allowing adequate time for rest, are very important. Walking, as you will see on p. 47, can be very helpful for morning sickness and be at the heart of your new daily routine.

Yoga in all its aspects, including the full Eight Limbs (set out in my book, ANCIENT WISDOM) and particularly the breathing and relaxation practices, will enable you to make the adjustment and to be aware of what your body needs. Your inner awareness is heightened at this time. Notice this new level of perception, as it will develop throughout your pregnancy and go on increasing in parenthood.

In this section I am giving a programme of relaxation, breathing and meditation only. They are particularly suitable now but remain good throughout pregnancy. If you are experienced and feel happy to continue doing postures, please go on to the next chapter for suggestions, but come back to this one for breathing and meditation as it is the beginning of a process which will go on through pregnancy and is described progressively in this book.

MIDWIFERY NOTES:

HORMONAL AND PHYSIOLOGICAL CHANGES IN THE FIRST TRIMESTER, WITH HELPFUL POSTURES

TIREDNESS

Tiredness at this stage is mainly due to the enormous change the body is undergoing with the fertilization of the embryo and the subsequent development of the yolk sac to maintain the embryo. The female hormones progesterone and oestrogen are increased to maintain the integrity of the embryo.

Yoga for tiredness
Meditation and relaxation.

THE UTERUS

By twelve weeks' gestation, the uterus is just above the symphisis pubis and is about the size of a grapefruit. The woman feels 'bloated', overweight with associated exhaustion of carrying extra bulk.

Yoga for this area
Relaxation and gentle *pranayama* (breathing).

BREASTS

The greatest changes to the breasts happen in the first thirteen weeks of pregnancy as many new ducts are formed then. The breasts may feel painful, large and tender to the touch. This is normal and is caused by the increased levels of the hormones progesterone and oestrogen,

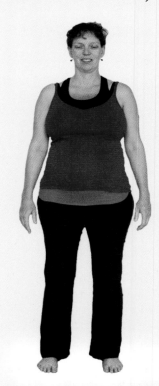

TADASANA (MOUNTAIN POSE)

which is stimulated by the development of the placenta.

Yoga for this area
Tadasana (Mountain pose, see photo on previous page), focusing on spreading the breastbone.

HEART RATE AND RESPIRATION

Because of the increased blood volume that allows for the extra demand the foetus is making on the body, the heart rate will increase from the seventh week of pregnancy onwards. The blood-pressure drops due to vasodilation in early pregnancy and in some women this can result in feeling faint, light-headed or indeed actually fainting. Increased heart rate and the effect of progesterone and oestrogen leads to some shortness of breath and increased blood volume can sometimes lead to nosebleeds.

Yoga for the heart
Relaxation, meditation and gentle awareness of the breath.

PRODUCTION OF URINE

The increase in passing urine and particularly at night are thought to be due to the pressure the growing uterus is exerting on the bladder and the resultant decrease in bladder capacity.

Yoga for the urinary system
Tadasana (Mountain pose, previous page).

NAUSEA AND SICKNESS

Again, the combination of hormonal changes and psychological changes are thought to be responsible for the feelings of nausea and vomiting in early pregnancy. Hunger also increases and small, frequent meals will help to maintain the body's blood sugar levels.

Yoga for nausea
Relaxation, meditation and gentle awareness of the breath, and *Tadasana* (Mountain pose, previous page).

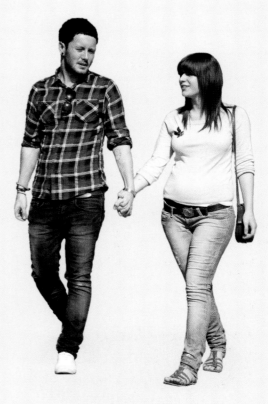

A GOOD WALK IN THE FRESH AIR WILL HELP TO ALLEVIATE NAUSEA

1. RELAXATION
WITH CALMING BREATH

Anapanasati is a Pali word that the Buddha used to denote awareness or mindfulness of the breath without altering it, so that the mind relaxes down to connect to the body and so becomes calm.

Lie down on the floor, futon or bed, with the heels extended gently and arms relaxed out to the side. If there is any strain under your back or knees, put a rolled up blanket under your knees as Emily has done in the photo. If it is more comfortable, also put your hands on your lower belly so you can feel more in touch with your baby.

Let your mind relax down into your body and become aware of your breath moving through it. Feel that every cell of your body can breathe, including all the cells of your growing baby.

Relax into this movement. Feel your back ribs spreading out from your spine. This means your diaphragms are moving to bring the breath in and out. Many of us breathe from only the top chest with the secondary respiratory muscles.

When you feel rested and restored, roll onto your side to come up to sitting.

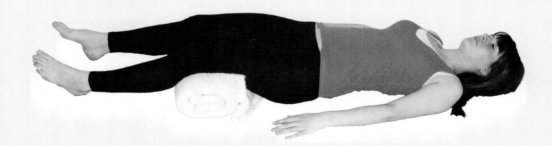

2. MARJARIASANA AND PINDASANA
BREATHING ON ALL FOURS (CAT POSE) AND CHILD POSE

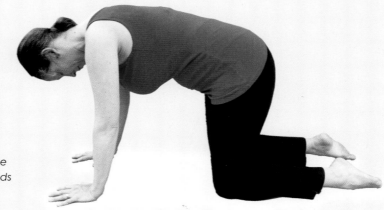

Points to watch*: ease the arms up into the shoulders to open across the chest and collarbone (sternum and clavicle). Lengthen the spine, and spread the hands down into the earth*

The photo shows Simone in Cat pose, which is suggested to help you feel the back and side ribs spread as you breathe, especially if you do not feel the breath in the back of the body very easily. In pregnancy and childbirth it is particularly important to breathe from the pelvic floor diaphragm and the thoracic diaphragm at the bottom of the ribs. This relaxes you and the foetus inside you and moves the whole body. Remember this awareness of breathing into the back of the body and the movement of the diaphragms in everyday life.

Come onto all fours as shown. Because of the different shape of the spine now, it is much easier to feel the breath moving the back and side ribs out, away from the spine. You can fill the spine up slightly, as Simone is doing, so that the ribs can open more. That lets the lungs move away from the spine as they fill with the breath, and lets the spine lengthen more out of the hips, and more through the shoulderblades as you exhale.

Then rest down into *Pindasana* (Child pose), shown overleaf.

When you have felt this movement of the breath, sit in a posture that's comfortable to you, rest against the wall or sit in a chair if you are tired or your back needs support. Let the mind rest down again to feel your breath moving through your body.

Now bring your awareness to the new life growing inside you. Connect to this life; maybe feel a pulsation or sense of life, light inside you.

In the first three to four months of my pregnancy I was aware of a sense of 'energy' dancing around me, then quite suddenly it was inside me. Is this what they call the quickening? It's then that I felt the movement of the baby. First I had this sense that the subtle celestial body of my baby (the *ananda maya kosa*, see Introduction, pp. 13–14) was moving around me.

Then, when she was ready to become more physical, I could feel her inside me.

If your mind wanders (which it will inevitably do as that's its nature) bring it gently back to your breath and your body.

Do this for as long as you feel able. To finish, take a couple of deeper breaths and bring your hands into *Namaste*, prayer position, if you wish to give thanks for the life inside you at the end of your meditation. This finishing in *Namaste* is traditional in yoga.

Points to wach: *keep the eyes and brain relaxed down. Note Simone's relaxed shoulders and her active feet and legs*

Points to watch: *take the shoulders back to lengthen the neck. Spread the ribs as you breathe, and rest the hips back and down on the heels. Rest the brow down on the earth, or on a block if the head is not naturally right down*

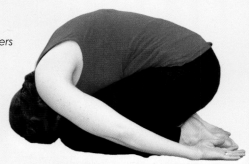

3. Trataka

MEDITATION ON THE MOON

The moon has long been a source of fascination and connection for many cultures, with its links to the feminine energy. This first trimester is a good time to link to the moon energy.

If you can sit outside without getting cold, or in a window with the moon in sight, this would be great. Otherwise visualize it, or use the picture here, or the one on p. 24. Be aware as you sit or stand of the phases of the moon, from new to full and back again. Feel the link with your cycle and to a woman's cycle from girlhood to menstruation to pregnancy to childbirth, and finally to the cessation of that cycle and transition into a 'wise woman'. Feel your place in that cycle. See the luminosity, brightness and clarity the moon gives.

Close your eyes and visualize the moon within you. It may be at the level of your heart, your womb, or your brow: just let that be.

Now let your awareness expand into your role within the whole planet called earth; your role in the eternal rhythm of birth, life, death and rebirth.

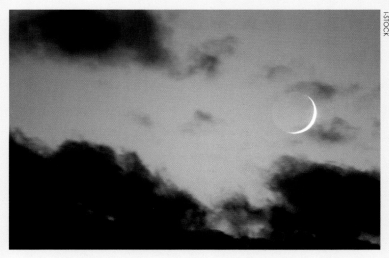

I-STOCK

51

THE KEY TO THE CORRECT CARRIAGE OF THE BODY AND TO THE HEALTH OF THE CHILD TO COME LIES IN THE FEET. A HEALTHY BODY PROVIDES THE FOUNDATION FOR THE MIND TO FUNCTION IN A WELL REGULATED DIRECTION. THE CHILD IN THE WOMB IS THE PRODUCT OF THE LIVING THOUGHT OF THE MOTHER THROUGHOUT HER PREGNANCY. THE HEALTHY BODY AND THE HEALTHY MIND OF THE WOULD-BE MOTHER PROVIDE THE FERTILE SOIL, FOR THE PHYSICAL, MENTAL AND SPIRITUAL GROWTH OF THE CHILD.

YOGA HELPS A MOTHER IN DELIVERING A ROBUST AND HEALTHY CHILD. IT KEEPS HER BODY TRIM AND LESSENS THE TENSION IN HER NERVES AND MIND BY TEACHING HER THE ART OF RELAXATION. ASANAS AND BREATHING EXERCISES BRING EXPANSION AND EXTENSION, SO THAT ROOM IS MADE IN THE MOTHER'S BELLY FOR THE CHILD TO KICK, STRETCH AND DESCEND. LABOUR PAINS BECOME BEARABLE AND DELIVERY IS NATURAL. IN PARTICULAR, THERE IS A SENSE OF FREEDOM AND JOY, A SENSE OF WARMTH AND LOVE.

SRI BKS IYENGAR

PREGNANCY IS A PRIVILEGE. A STATE OF GRACE. IT IS A WOMAN'S GREATEST, DEEPEST EXPERIENCE. WATCH — LET US SEE THE FIRE CATCH AND THEN BLAZE FROM POSTURE TO POSTURE. WATCH THE EYES, THEIR INTENSITY, THIS DIVINE GLOW THAT BEGINS TO RADIATE AND SHINE. DAWN! A HUMAN BEING EXPRESSING DIVINITY.

DR FREDERICK LEBOYER

BOTH OF THESE EXTRACTS ARE DERIVED FROM THE BOOK INNER BEAUTY, INNER LIGHT BY DR FRANCIS LEBOYER AND ITS PREFACE BY SRI BKS IYENGAR

3. The Second Trimester: Four to Six Months

 THE SECOND trimester represents a new stage, when the body has adjusted to being pregnant. After ten weeks the placenta and placental hormones are fully functional, so that the baby's system is settled, with the result that by twelve to fourteen weeks we may feel much better in ourselves – with more energy, more vitality. The nausea usually goes and we enjoy life again.

There follows a sequence of postures that can be practised during this period, with appropriate precautions.

On pp 73–7 are Sally's notes on any problems you might have and yoga that would help with these specific issues. Your yoga practice will increase and enhance that feeling of wellbeing and blooming that you can see in pregnant women in the second trimester, when their complexion is radiant and their whole being radiates joy and amazement at this wonderful event taking place within their body.

Your legs will need to be strengthened and firmed to carry your baby. The standing postures suggested will give strength and endurance for the changes in life and body, including carrying the extra weight, and will open up the pelvis ready for labour.

In our Western bodies our legs do not always sustain us very well: they have weakened from our sitting in chairs, car seats, and our more sedentary lifestyle. Before they had cars, many people would walk miles every day. In this trimester, walking for at least thirty minutes a day is generally recommended.

PRECAUTIONS FOR THIS TRIMESTER

1. Always keep the abdominal area open and unrestricted, so do not practise postures such as those twists where the twist is across the body. In sitting twists, keep the spine lengthened forward and up, or use a chair or wall as shown in the next chapter, so the baby is never restricted. Suitable twists are *Bharadvajasana* (p. 87) and sitting postures such as cross-legged and Hero. All these are shown in the next chapter, on the third trimester.

2. Do not practise standing twists, such as Reverse Triangle pose.

3. Keep the spine lengthened forward in all standing postures, as shown in Tripod pose (*Prasarita padottanasana*, p. 62).

4. Make sure in all postures that you are not under any strain across your abdomen or with your breathing.

5. If you take your arms over your head, do not hold them there, and if you feel any rush of blood to your face, bring the arms down immediately and sit down. Do not do postures with arms overhead after that.

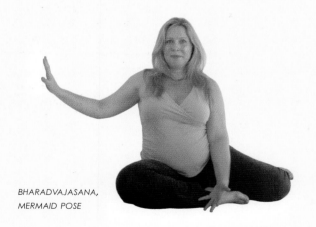

BHARADVAJASANA, MERMAID POSE

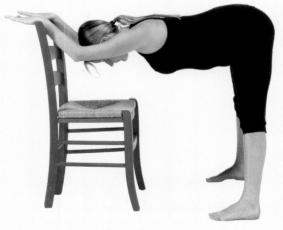

PRASARITA PADOTTANASANA TRIPOD POSE, WITH A CHAIR

1. UTKATASANA
'CHAIR' POSE, USING THE WALL, AND GOING INTO
TADASANA (MOUNTAIN POSE)

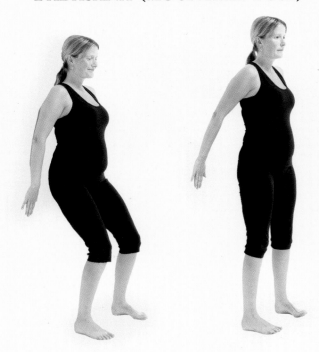

Utkatanasana literally means 'Fierce' or 'Ardent' pose but it is often translated as 'Chair pose'.

Stand with your back against a wall, with the knees directly over the ankles and arms spreading into the wall, and the back rested on the wall, as Angela is doing in the lefthand picture. This will help to spread the sacrum back so that the increasing weight of the baby does not bring the whole centre of gravity too far forward. (This needs to happen to an extent, but if it is too much, it will create too much lordosis in the lumbar spine, and

so cause strain in the back and sacroiliac joints.)

Let your baby relax back in your pelvis. Spread your upper back, lengthen your tailbone down, and then take your hands onto the wall and gently ease yourself away to standing (righthand picture). As you do this keep the feeling of resting more into your back body, and feel the lengthening up through your spine from your tailbone.

This posture lengthens the spine and spreads the sacrum.

55

2. Parsvottanasana
EXTENDED SIDE STRETCH OR EGRET POSE

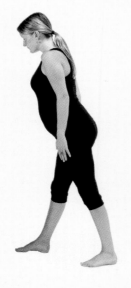 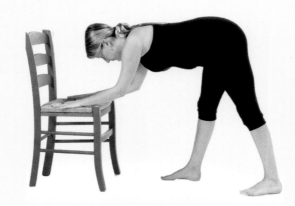 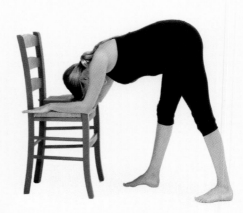

The literal translation of *Parsvottan-asana* is 'sideways forward bend', but I like to call this pose 'Egret' as it reminds me of how egrets stand, lifted up through their legs into their

hips. Place a chair in front of you.

From *Tadasana*, Mountain pose, step one foot forward (first picture). Go down firmly through your heels to move your spine forward, so

that your hands and wrists rest on the chair (second picture).

Lengthen your legs firmly up into the hip joint, as your heels spread down, to relax your spine forward

and rest your head on the chair (third picture).

From here you can go into either Triangle pose or full *Parsvottanasana*: see next page.

3. Utthita Trikonasana and Full Parsvottanasana
stretched triangle pose and sideways forward bend (egret pose)

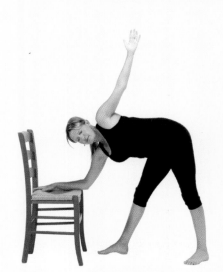
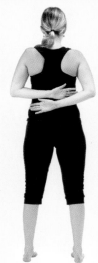
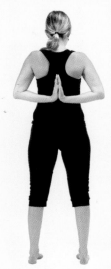
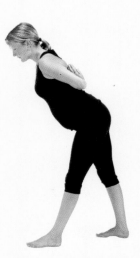

From 'Egret' you can go on into Triangle (lefthand picture). Keep the arm on the same side as the forward leg resting down, and turn the toes of the back leg out. Lengthen up through the thighbone to open the hip of the back leg, so that the spine spirals around on its axis towards the ceiling and the ribs open – and maybe the arm extends up, as shown in the first picture. To come out, spread firmly down through your back foot to lift up through your hips and bring you up. Change to the other side.

To go on to full *Parsvottanasana*, from *Tadasana* rest your hands across your back so that your shoulderblades and shoulder joints broaden out (second picture). Spreading from the inner edge of the scapula (shoulderblade) bring the hands together in *Parsva namaste* (Prayer position behind).

Then, stepping forward, lengthen up through the thigh bone into the hip joint to take the spine forward and up (right). To come up, spread firmly into the back heel to bring the spine back up and step forward to do the other side.

4. VRKSASANA
TREE POSE

Lightly rest your fingers on the wall. Spread firmly down through one heel, lifting the other heel and bringing that knee right up above your hip to open it out. Spread your foot firmly into your opposite thigh. Open your arms to the side and spread into the back ribs.

If you feel steady, bring your hands together in *Namaste*, as in the right-hand picture.

Change to the other side.

This pose calms and steadies the whole system, moves the hips, and lengthens and strengthens the legs and spine.

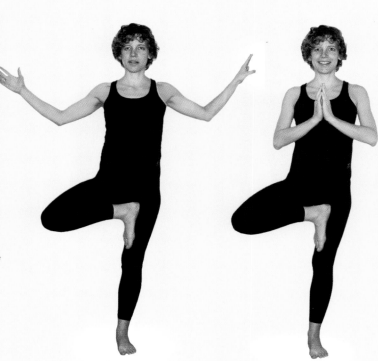

Points to watch: *lengthen up the leg from the foot so that the hip is not jammed. Make sure that the upper heel is lifted firmly into the hip joint, while the heel on which you are standing spreads firmly down*

5. HAND ONTO THE WALL
HAND INTO THE WALL

Standing sideways to the wall and keeping the shoulders soft, take the near hand at shoulder height onto the wall. This elbow should be slightly bent so that the shoulders do not stiffen. Maintain an awareness in the feet to keep the hips parallel and facing forward.

Spreading the palm of the hand into the wall, feel how that frees the whole arm, frees it deep into the armpit, and how it also lifts and opens the chest, freeing the breath.

Lift the heel of the hand to lengthen the fingers onto the wall and dome the palm of the hand. Then, keeping the contact there, let the heel of the hand come down onto the wall.

Root the index finger firmly into

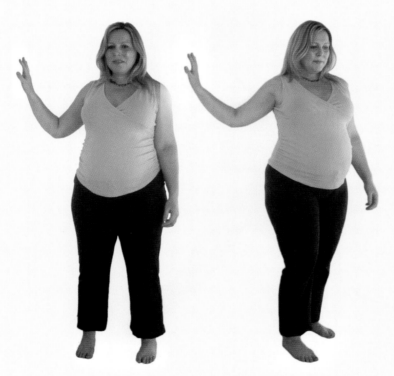

the wall to feel how that moves and frees, deeply, from the collar bone, and then – rooting down through the other fingers one by one – feel how that moves all around the shoulders to free the neck, upper arm and release deeply into the shoulder girdle.

Now turn the feet and whole body out into the room as shown right, keeping the back relaxed back, to open across the collarbone and breastbone more. Then come back to take the arm down. As you bring the arm down, feel the deep release that gives, and then go on to the other side.

This pose relaxes the shoulders and eases out strain in the neck. It helps with carpal tunnel problems (see Sally's notes on problems that could occur in the second trimester, p. 73).

6. VIRABHADRASANA I
WARRIOR I POSE

From *Tadasana*, Mountain pose, place your hands on the crest of your hips. Take a firm, dynamic step forward, bending the front knee directly above the ankle joint. Let the back heel lift to bring the hip of the back leg in line with the hip of the front leg.

Then, maintaining the forward movement of the hip, take the heel back towards the ground, moving the thigh bone into the hip joint to work the legs. Spread firmly down into both heels to free the hips, so that the spine lengthens up out of the hips. If there is any strain on the back, ease the spine further forward out of the hips, and go down through the heels more to bring life to the legs.

To move to the other side, step the back foot forward, going back to *Tadasana*, and then step

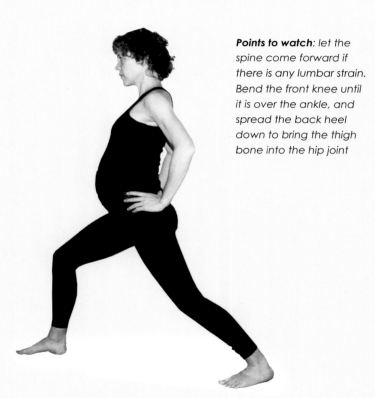

Points to watch: *let the spine come forward if there is any lumbar strain. Bend the front knee until it is over the ankle, and spread the back heel down to bring the thigh bone into the hip joint*

forward on that foot.

This pose is traditionally practised with the arms overhead. During pregnancy, however, if the arms are held overhead for any length of time there is a tendency for the blood-pressure to go up and the heart (which is working very hard anyway to develop and grow the baby) to feel under strain. This is even more likely in the third trimester. You would however feel pressure in the head if this were happening, and it may feel comfortable to swing the arms forward and up overhead, relaxing the shoulders down and moving the spine up through the shoulderblades. Then bring them down, so as not to hold them in this position.

This pose wakes up the hips and legs and strengthens the spine.

7. Ardha Chandrasana
HALF MOON POSE

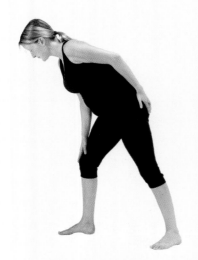
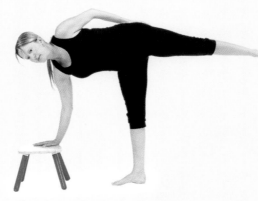

From standing, step one foot forward, firm the heel back, and lengthen into the thighs so that the spine comes forward, as in the first picture. Take your hand down onto the blocks or a firm stool.

Spread down into the standing heel and up into the hip joint to lift the back leg (second and third photos).

To come out of the pose, bend the standing leg to take the lifted leg down. Now change to the other side. If you feel unsure of yourself in this pose have your back against the wall. This will also open the hips more.

8. Prasarita Padottanasana
TRIPOD POSE

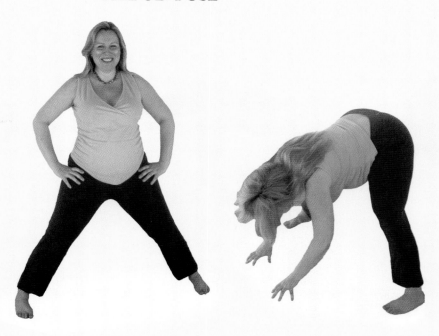

Points to watch:
spread firmly down through the heels, spreading the toes, so that the thighbone lifts into the hip joint and so lifts the pelvis off the thighs, making room for the baby

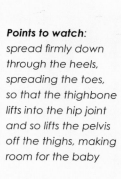

From standing, take your feet wide apart, and place your hands where thighs meet hips (as Joy is doing in the first photo).

From the hips, take the spine forward and down. If it is comfortable to do so, place the hands on the floor (second photo) or have a low stool or the seat of a chair in front of you. Angela demonstrates the use of the chair in the photographs opposite.

By the time you are in the third trimester you will need this chair all the more. Relax the head and let the spine come forward and down. This is especially helpful if your blood-pressure goes up, or the head is busy or aches.

Rest a moment or two, breathing into the back of your ribs. Spread firmly down through your feet to come up.

This pose lets the sacrum spread and hips open. All of these standing poses prepare the pelvis well for labour and childbirth, and strengthen the legs for carrying the baby both *in utero* and out of it.

This differs from the next pose in the position of the feet.

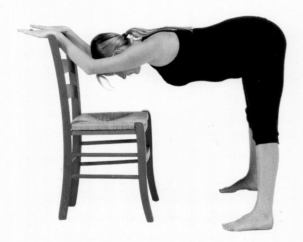
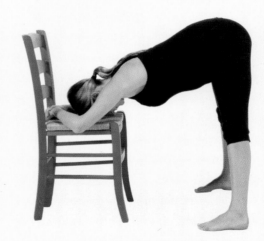

9. Uttanasana
STANDING FORWARD BEND, USING A CHAIR

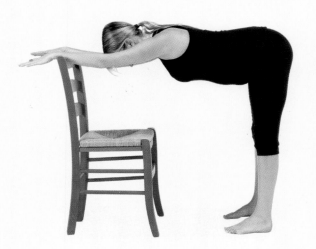 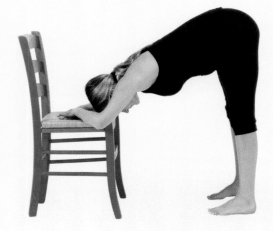

Stand near to a chair with the seat of the chair facing you and your feet just wider than hip width apart. Place your hands lightly on the back of the chair, then walk backwards until your spine is parallel to the floor. Your hands may then want to come down onto the seat of the chair as shown. Do not restrict the baby in any way. Relax there as long as is comfortable.

When you are ready to come up, walk back in towards the chair, so that you are coming out of it the way you went into it.

10. MALASANA
GARLAND POSE OR SQUAT

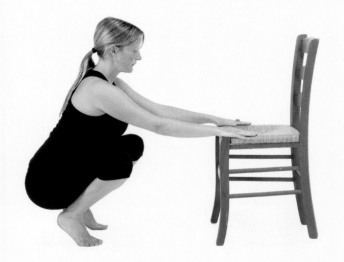

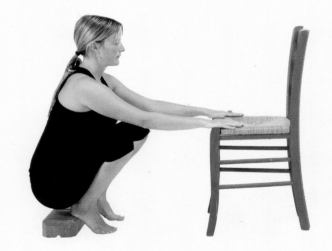

Sitting postures are included in the third trimester, chapter 4, as they are best when you are tired or when the blood-pressure tends to be elevated, but they can equally be practised in the sec-

ond trimester, so you could go on to those now or on to *Malasana*.

From *Uttanasana,* on the previous page, bend your knees so that you are squatting, as in the lefthand picture below. Let

your hips come down and your head lift up. Let the heels lift, as this wakes up the feet, especially the arches. Keeping the lift of the arches, the heels could lift over and down, as though there is a

stick under your arches, towards the ground or onto a block as shown in the righthand photo.

If this is at all a strain, or if you have backache, then use the wall, gradually sliding down as in the sequence of pictures below, until the hips are just lifted off the ground. If you go right down (as in the third picture), use the blocks as shown, or take the feet nearer to the wall.

NB: do not go down into a full squat after thirty-two weeks as it pushes the baby's head down too much into the head of the cervix (so you only go part of the way down into a squat) – until you are in labour, when it is good to do.

You could then rest down in *Baddha konasana*, Cobbler pose, against the wall, to relax and meditate (final picture), or go on into Dog pose, *Adho mukha svanasana*, opposite.

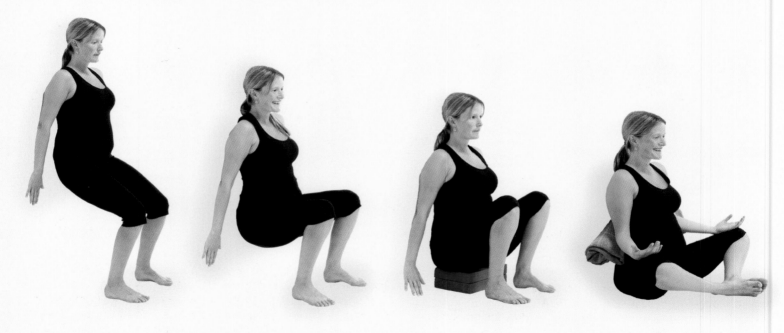

11. ADHO MUKHA SVANASANA
FACE-DOWN DOG POSE

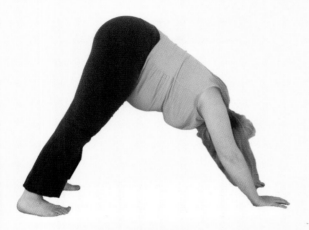

Points to watch: bring the spine forward through the shoulderblades, and ease the heels into the wall

Points to watch: spread into your sacrum and keep the shoulders spread out. Relax the knees and ease them away from one another to leave space for the baby

From Cat pose on all fours (p. 49), tuck your toes under and spread up and back through your heels to lift straight up so your spine comes forward and down, copying Joy in the lefthand picture. Spread down through your hands to broaden your shoulders and back ribs and lift up into your sacrum and then lengthen over and down into your heels. If there is any strain down through the arms, have your heels so that they are resting down and back against the wall as Panna is doing in the righthand picture.

Come down when ready, resting your head to the ground in *Pindasana*, Child pose, knees easing out to make space for the baby.

12. Viparita Karani
REVERSING ATTITUDE

Lie with your legs up the wall. Bend your knees and spread your feet into the wall to lift your pelvis, and now put a bolster – or one or two blocks or cushions – underneath your sacrum as shown, so that your tailbone rolls over the edge of them. This relaxes your tummy back and spreads your chest area out.

This should feel very comfortable; if there is any discomfort or pressure anywhere, especially in the neck or back, do not stay in the posture. Some women are more comfortable without the blocks.

IMPORTANT: to come out of this posture, take the bolster or blocks away first then roll over onto your side to come up to sitting.

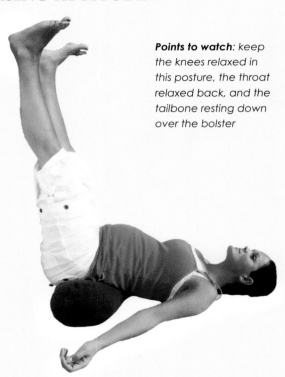

Points to watch: keep the knees relaxed in this posture, the throat relaxed back, and the tailbone resting down over the bolster

13. HALASANA AND SALAMBA SARVANGASANA
PLOUGH POSE AND SHOULDERSTAND

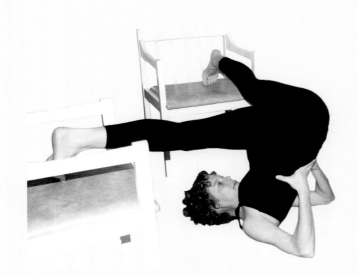

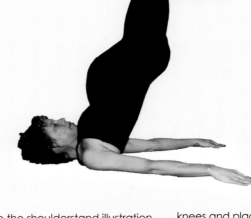

If *Viparita karani* (previous page) feels comfortable and beneficial to do, then you might like to try going over into *Halasana*, Plough pose, done with two chairs placed apart behind you to put your feet onto, as in the first photo. Lift up through

your legs so that your hips lift above your shoulders and heels extend away to bring feet onto the chair.

From this position you can lift up one leg at a time into Shoulderstand, especially if you did it before you were pregnant.

See the shoulderstand illustration overleaf, lefthand picture. Make sure you are not feeling any strain at all across your neck, back or tummy in this position.

If it's more comfortable, from the feet-on-chair position bend your

knees and place the feet against the wall. Spread the knees into the wall and lengthen your knees up towards the ceiling, so that your back lifts off the ground as shown – but only go so high as is comfortable for your neck and head.

Spread your arms and hands into the ground, to spread your shoulders and lift your upper back.

Do not stay in any of these positions if there is any pressure in the head, neck or throat. When it feels to be enough, relax

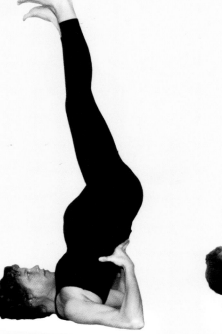

back down, using the hands to balance you into the ground and your feet into the wall, for a gentle landing – or alternatively bring your feet back onto the chairs and gently roll your back down, resting there.

These poses tone up all the internal organs, relieve any pressure on back and hips, and refresh and revitalize the whole body. Do not do them if there is any strain in your head, neck, back or abdomen. If there is, stay

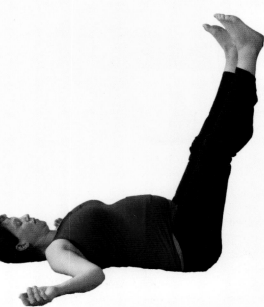

with the support in *Setu bandha sarvangasana*. Bridge pose (p. 34), or legs up the wall in *Urdhva dandasana*, Upside-down Staff pose, as Karen is doing (below right and p. 90). They also help to prevent varicose veins.

14. SAVASANA
RELAXATION

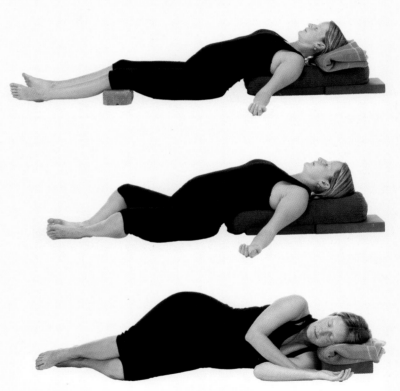

As your baby grows, you will find it gradually less comfortable to lie flat on your back. Find enough bolsters, cushions, etc to make it comfortable to stretch out (top and middle photographs). If it is still not comfortable, then lie on your side (bottom picture).

The moment when it feels uncomfortable may come while you are doing it, or it may come afterwards, as the baby can be pushed up and restrict the blood supply to the placenta. You will certainly need to start elevating the back from around four months.

You can bring the feet together in *Supta badha konasana* (Lying-down Cobbler pose, middle picture) but don't let there be any strain in your hips. It does free the hips if it is comfortable. If your pelvis tilts up, or your back is at all uncomfortable, put some lift under your knees.

Extending the exhalation

As you relax, bring your awareness right down through your body, and feel the baby resting back. (Be ready for the discovery that babies can sometimes get active in this pose, however, as they have more room!)

Feel the breath in the back of your body. Then, gently inhaling, go with the exhalation so that it lengthens gradually with each breath. See if you have a sense of going into the exhalation and then waiting for your breath to come in when it's ready. Feel the natural pause at the end of the exhalation.

Continue this for as long as it feels comfortable and the mind stays with the movements of your breath. Then let your breath come back to normal before rolling onto your side to come up to sitting.

This gentle extension of the exhalation will help greatly in labour and childbirth, as it will enable you to go with the contractions and the passage of the baby down the birth canal. It is good preparation for Viloma, which follows.

IN THIS BODY, IN THIS TOWN OF SPIRIT, THERE IS A LITTLE HOUSE SHAPED LIKE A LOTUS, AND IN THAT HOUSE THERE IS A LITTLE SPACE.
ONE SHOULD KNOW WHAT IS THERE.
WHAT IS THERE? WHY IS IT SO IMPORTANT?
THERE IS AS MUCH IN THAT LITTLE SPACE WITHIN THE HEART, AS THERE IS IN THE WHOLE WORLD OUTSIDE.
HEAVEN, EARTH, FIRE, WIND, SUN, MOON, LIGHTNING, STARS; WHATEVER IS AND WHATEVER IS NOT, EVERYTHING IS THERE.
CHHANDOGYA UPANISHAD, BOOK EIGHT, TRANS. ALISTAIR SHEARER AND PETER RUSSELL

---

15. VILOMA
LADDER BREATH, SITTING OR LYING

The *Viloma* breath follows on from the extending of the exhalation in *Savasana*. It is a good idea to practise that first for a few sessions before going on to this one, if you have not done much *pranayama* (awareness of the breath) before.

After a few breaths of extending the exhalation, inhale, and then as you exhale pause, and then exhale again. Do not hold on: exhale again whenever you are ready, pause again, and exhale again until you feel the breath has gone right out, so that it feels as though there is a comma in the cycle, a very brief pause. Then let it come easily in.

Continue with this as long as your awareness stays with it. It does not matter how many pauses there are on the exhalation as long as there is no strain.

When it feels enough *Viloma*, without any strain, sit and feel the effect of it, perhaps contemplating the above passage from the Upanishads. The pauses can also be put into the inhalation, as that lifts your energy. Pausing on the exhalation calms your energy and is generally more suited to pregnancy and labour than pausing on the inhalation, however.

This *pranayama* will assist labour by allowing you to go with contractions more easily, as well as bringing relaxation and ease of breathing generally. It is also helpful for insomnia.

MIDWIFERY NOTES
WITH HELPFUL POSTURES

Most women feel very well, healthy and 'blooming' at this stage of pregnancy. However there are some problems that could occur, including the following.

NERVOUS SYSTEM

Carpal tunnel syndrome, caused by oedema (swelling) on the median nerves in the wrist.

The major anatomical and physiological changes come as a direct result of hormonal changes, particularly in the hormone progesterone which causes relaxation of smooth muscle throughout the body.

Yoga postures
Hand on the wall (right – for instructions, see p. 59).

Namaste, with the hands at

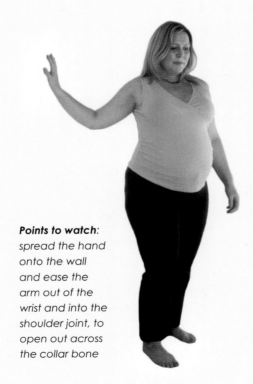

Points to watch:
spread the hand onto the wall and ease the arm out of the wrist and into the shoulder joint, to open out across the collar bone

breastbone level, and then moving to place them lightly on the head. Then, thirdly, spreading the arms to the side, unpeeling the fingers and hands gradually. Finally, bring one hand onto the other forearm and ease the forearm out from the wrist as though you were putting on a long, tight evening glove, extending the fingers away, out of their joints.

All standing postures, done facing the wall and with hands on the wall a few inches higher than the shoulders, making sure the elbows are releasing down.

Uttanasana (Standing forward bend) and *Prasarita padottanasana* (Tripod pose) using a chair (see pp. 62–4).

SKIN CHANGES

Corticosteroid levels increase, which can lead to the development of striae gravidarum (stretch marks).

DIGESTIVE SYSTEM

There is a marked reduction of gastric and intestinal tone, and progesterone causes the cardiac sphincter at the entrance to the stomach to relax. This can result in indigestion and heartburn. These in turn can be aggravated by the enlarging uterus.

The smooth muscle of the bowel can become sluggish, resulting in constipation and haemorrhoids (piles).

For some women, there is a change in taste and smell of some foods and drinks. For instance, coffee and fried foods may become unpalatable and their smell can cause nausea. This obviously is a sign that your body does not want whatever is causing such a reaction.

Yoga postures
Bharadvajasana (Mermaid pose) using a chair in front to put hand on (see third trimester), *Dandasana* (Staff pose: see third trimester), *Janu sirsasana* (see third trimester, and use a chair if it is needed), *Baddha konasana* (Cobbler pose: see third trimester), *Adho Mukha Svanasana* (Dog pose, p. 67), *Viparita Karani* (p. 68),

supported *Halasana* (Plough pose, p. 69). Make sure there is no strain in the face.

CARDIOVASCULAR SYSTEM

By the end of the second trimester, the cardiac output can increase by up to 40% to supply the ever-increasing blood vessels to the uterus and the enlarging placenta. There is also an increase in plasma volume of up to 50% which decreases the viscosity of the blood and improves capillary flow particularly to perfuse (supply) the growing foetus and placenta.

Progesterone acts on the smooth muscle of the blood vessels, decreasing their elasticity and causing them to relax everywhere, but it could manifest as swollen ankles, for example; this vasodilation can lead to the feeling of faintness and light-headedness. Another effect of the increase in plasma volume is haemodilution which can manifest itself as anaemia which causes women to feel tired and lethargic.

Another effect of an increase in plasma volume is loss of fluid out of the capillaries resulting in generalized oedema (puffiness).

Supine hypotension (low blood-pressure when lying flat).

Posture can have a major effect on blood-pressure and the supine position (lying flat on the back) can decrease cardiac output by as much as 25% because of compression of the inferior vena cava, the blood vessel that takes the deoxygenated blood back to the heart, by the ever-enlarging uterus.

Yoga postures
Anapanasati (calming breathing, see p. 48) in all postures and all activities.

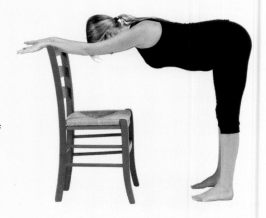

Uttanasana, Standing forward bend and Tripod pose using a chair (see picture left and p. 63).

Moving slowly from one posture to another, especially where the head is down, will help adjust blood-pressure.

Supta virasana (p. 27), Supta baddha konasana (p. 71), Malasana (p. 65). All need to be well supported.

Savasana (relaxation) and meditation, chanting Om.

Hridaya mudra. For this, bring the index finger right in to the root of the thumb, then bring the thumb to touch the middle two fingers. See picture below; more details in next chapter. The index finger represents the ego consciousness, the thumb the heart consciousness, the middle fingers the mind. So in the heart

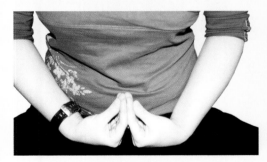

mudra we are reining the ego and then connecting the mind to the heart.

RESPIRATORY SYSTEM

Progesterone and oestrogen cause the respiratory centre to be more sensitive to carbon dioxide. This can influence the breathing, forcing the woman to breathe more consciously or become short of breath.

Blood volume expansion can result in swelling of the upper respiratory mucosa, leading to nasal congestion and sometimes nosebleeds.

The enlarging uterus can cause the diaphragm to be elevated by as much as 4 cm, resulting in the ribcage being displaced upwards and the lung capacity becoming reduced by as much as 5%. Sometimes called 'flaring of the ribs', this is usually annoying rather than debilitating.

Yoga postures
Utkatasana, standing squat against a wall, breathing into back of the body, followed by *Tadasana*, breathing into the back body (see photo at right).

Baddha konasana (Cobbler pose: see

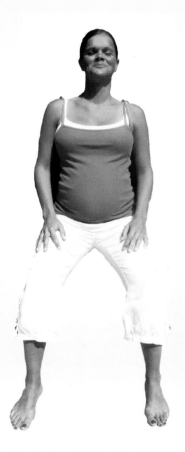

UTKATASANA

p. 88), with back against a wall.

All postures need to be done breathing more into back of lungs to take pressure off the front and to calm the whole system. They should be followed by *Anapanasati* (calming breath) in *Savasana* and in sitting.

MUSCULOSKELETAL SYSTEM

Oestrogen, progesterone and relaxin all influence the joints, the connective tissue and the ligaments at this stage of pregnancy. Oestrogen makes connective tissue more pliable, causing the joint capsules to relax and the pelvic joints to become more mobile. Progesterone relaxes and weakens the ligaments, while relaxin softens the pelvic ligaments and joints in preparation for labour. This is all working towards making the pelvis larger for delivery of the foetus.

Other results are often a change in stature, and backache. At this time the posture alters to accommodate the enlarging womb and an increasing lordosis shifts a women's centre of gravity back over her legs. This and an increasing

mobility of the pelvis joints (the sacroilliac and sacrococcygeal joints) may explain the waddling gait of many heavily pregnant women and the lower back pain experienced.

Yoga postures
Backache: *Utkatasana* against wall. *Tadasana*, Mountain, bringing the centre of gravity back by moving iliac crests back.

Adho mukha svanasana (Dog pose, p. 67 and above right) with heels into the wall. Standing asanas using the wall or chair.

Sitting asanas using chair as for pre-eclampsia.

Malasana, Garland pose or squat (p. 65).

Pindasana (Child or Embryo pose, below right, and see p. 29 or p. 136), with knees wide and using a chair or blocks, or on ball.

Savasana (relaxation, p. 71) with legs resting on chair in the first eighteen weeks. After about eighteen weeks, or if this is more comfortable generally, place a blanket or bolster under the knees and upper back.

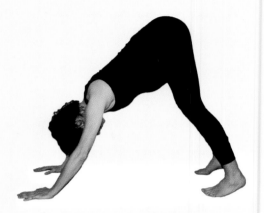

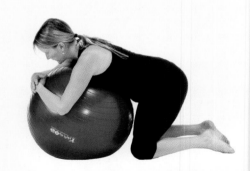

*ADHO MUKHA SVANASANA AND
PINDASANA OVER A BALL*

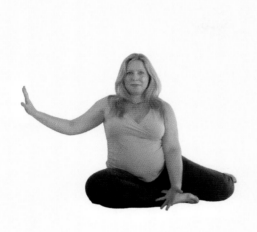
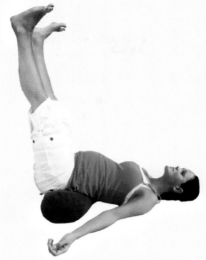

BHARADVAJASANA AND
VIPARITA KARANI

URINARY SYSTEM

Progesterone also influences the ureters (the tubes leading to the kidneys) by relaxing them, and sometimes urine can 'pool' in the now U-shaped tube, and the pregnant woman is thus more predisposed to urinary tract infections. This can sometimes manifest as backache too.

Stress incontinence can affect some women as a result of the relaxing effect of progesterone on the internal urethral sphincter and the pressure on the bladder of the ever-increasing uterus.

Yoga postures
Practice *Mula bandha mudra* (see p. 141) gently, in all asanas.

Bharadvajasana (Mermaid pose, p. 83 and left), *Viparita Karani* (reversing attitude, p. 68 and right), *Salamba*

Sirsasana (supported headstand, p. 101), but only if you have practised it regularly before becoming pregnant.

Salamba sarvangasana (Shoulderstand, p. 69), using chairs or wall, again only if well practised before pregnancy.

NB: in all twists, make sure there is no compression in the abdomen; and in inverted poses. no flushing in the face.

4. The Third Trimester: Seven to Nine Months

SEVEN to nine months is the time when we begin to want to slow down and relax more. Remember, pregnancy is like walking up a hill that gets steeper and steeper. All your vital organs are working much harder to build the baby's systems, even when you are at rest.

So listen to your body and your baby's needs. Listen to how you are feeling and how you can tune into how your baby is responding. In the last month it is particularly helpful template event place to rest and continue this wonderful that is taking in you.

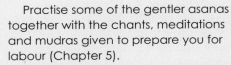

Practise some of the gentler asanas together with the chants, meditations and mudras given to prepare you for labour (Chapter 5).

Here are some postures that can be practised any time in pregnancy if your body feels like it, so long as there is no nausea and they do not make you very tired. They are especially helpful in this later stage.

1. Hip Moving

This movement and rotation of the hips, described by student Marielle Churaqui, will help in all stages of pregnancy from fourteen weeks on and in labour, but it is good to do beforehand. It is particularly helpful if the baby is in breech (upside-down so that feet or bottom will come out first) or occipital posterior (OP: around the wrong way, so that the back of the head, the occiput, is towards the spine, i.e. posterior).

Marielle describes this movement as 'best done standing, leaning forward with the hands resting on a wall or on any sort of support such as a windowsill. The hands can be either at shoulder level or much lower – whatever feels comfortable, but the knees must be kept soft. Alternatively, the hip movement can be done bending over a chair with hands on it and the feet firm, or in Cat pose, or over a ball. See the photographs below and opposite for some of the various possibilities. If you use Cat pose, care needs to be taken to keep the centre of balance towards the hips rather than over-loading the shoulders.

Gently swinging and circling the hips, or describing a figure of eight or a circle with the hips, can help the baby engage if the movement is practised regularly. These hip movements are beneficial throughout pregnancy as they soften the pelvic floor in preparation for the birth. They also gently massage the abdominal area and the lower back.

This may be the reason they seem to encourage breech babies to turn. They help to take the baby into the optimal position for the birth. Moving the tail of the spine back and forth also seems to encourage the baby to move downward and engage. Many women also find these rhythmic movements very soothing during labour as they can alleviate pain in the back.

Photos below show the movement done with a ball, when it is nice to rest your head down after.

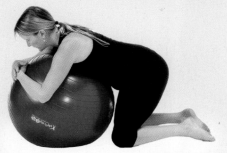
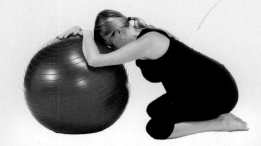

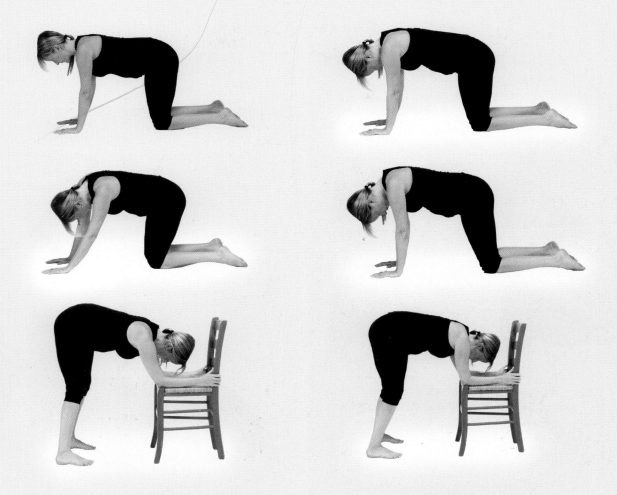

2. SUPPORTED VIRASANA AND SUPTA VIRASANA
HERO POSE AND EXTENDING-THE-SPINE-BACKWARDS HERO

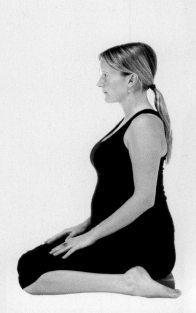

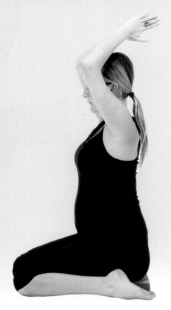

picture, and spread your thighs back into your sacrum. That will lengthen your spine, straight up. Gather your arms back into your shoulder joint so that your shoulders broaden. Now spread down into your feet and back into your thighs, so that your arms lift from under your ribs, where the muscles for the arms begin, as shown in the righthand photo. In this way you will not tighten, and instead lift from your shoulder. The shoulders will then rest back into *Supta Virasana* as shown.

Now arrange enough support behind to lie back comfortably, as Joy is doing in the photograph below, so that there is no strain on your knees or feet. Then let your spine lengthen up out of your hips and gently ease first into one hip then the other.

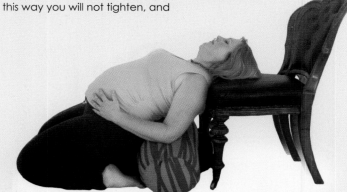

Kneel down with at least one block or cushion between your feet. It is important to have some lift under your buttock bones, even if you did not need it before you were pregnant, as otherwise the pubic bone and base area are too pushed down, as in the squat.

Rest your hands on your thighs, as Angela is doing in the lefthand

So long as your back feels comfortable, rest back onto the support and relax there, gently aware of your breath.

Feel how this pose gives a lot of space for you to breathe easily, especially into the back ribs, and also gives space for the baby to move. Stay there just as long as feels comfortable. Do not let there be any strain in your back at all.

When you are ready to come up, place your hands on your feet and lift your head and your breastbone by taking your hands firmly down, spreading up into your shoulders so that the whole spine comes up as one. Rest forward in *Pindasana*, Child pose (as Karen demonstrates, below left). Then come onto all fours, gently stretching your legs out one after the other behind you (below right).

This pose rests and restores tired legs. It relaxes and helps to spread the sacrum, frees the hips and spine and opens the diaphragm so you can breathe more easily. It also helps to open the pelvic floor for birth.

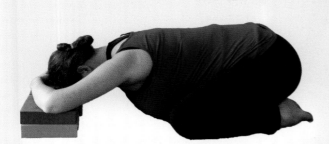

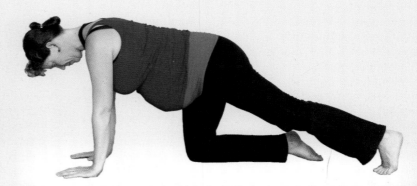

3. Upavistha Konasana
WIDE ANGLE POSE

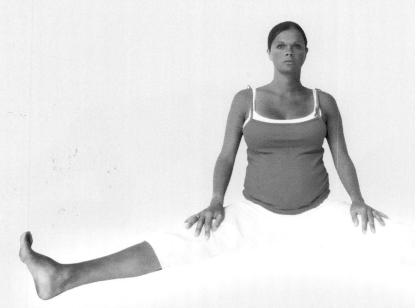

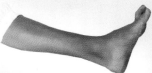

Points to watch: *don't try and stretch too wide with the legs. Spread down into the hells, and spread down, too, through the pubic bone.*

Sit with your legs out wide, as Saskia is demonstrating, lengthening your spine up and spreading your fingertips down or onto thighs as shown, so that you feel the easing out of your legs and an opening across your sacrum and heart area. Use your fingertips, spreading into the floor, to spread your shoulders and collar bone so that your thoracic spine (upper back) can move

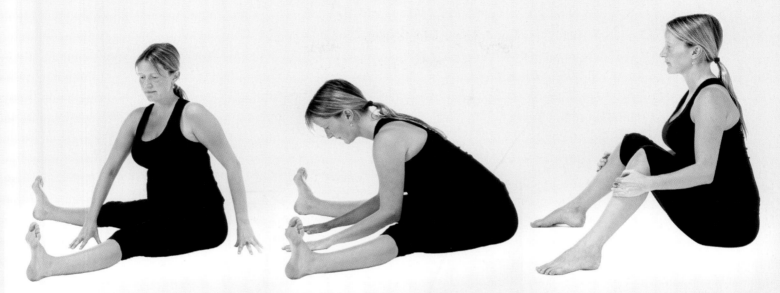

forward and up through your shoulderblades.

To turn over your left leg as Angela is doing above, spread back from your right heel to the hip so that the spine twists on its axis, spreading the fingers either side of the left leg. Repeat over the right leg.

Now come to the centre, and spread your fingers forward to bring the whole spine forward.

Spread back from your heels into your hip joint. Keep the spine forward and up so the baby is not squashed and the spine carries on waking up and lengthening.

To come up, spread back into your sacrum and bend the knees, to take the feet firmly down (righthand photo).

This pose opens the pelvic floor for birth and extends the legs and spine.

4. Janu Sirsasana
HEAD TO KNEE POSE

This is literally 'head-to-knee pose' but there is more extension of the spine if it stays forward and up. It is particularly helpful during pregnancy to use a chair, as Angela demonstrates, so that the baby is not constricted in any way.

It also relieves back strain, tiredness, headache or high blood-pressure. It does actually give more movement to your spine and hips to use the chair so do not think of it as just an easy option.

From the last posture, Wide angle pose, bend one leg so that your foot is turned upwards near the opposite thigh. Place your hands on the chair or ground, extending and then spiralling your spine on its axis around towards the straight leg. Then ease forward from your hips so that you can rest your head and arms on the chair as shown. Stay there as long as you find it comfortable.

Repeat the pose on the other side. For high blood-pressure or pre-eclampsia, it is helpful to stay on each side for between two and four minutes.

***Points to watch**: lengthen the spine up and spread the thigh into the hip joint. Spread into the heels, and spread the shoulders when you move into the position resting on the chair. Rest the head down*

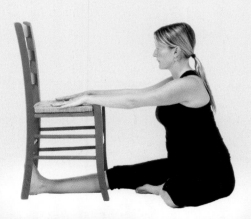
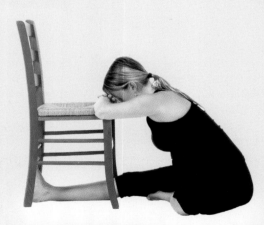

5. BHARADVAJASANA
MERMAID POSE

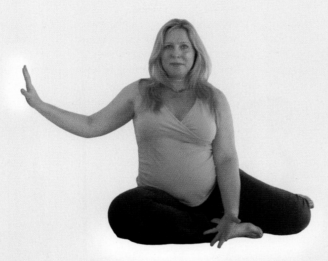

Points to watch: *spread the hand onto the wall, and ease the spine up and out of hips to spiral it around on its axis, towards the wall*

From *Janu sirsasana*, take one leg around behind you as in Hero pose (p. 82), but leave the other as it was, putting a hand on the wall like Joy is doing here. This encourages you to lengthen up out of the hips more in order to spiral the spine around over the front leg. Repeat on other side. This posture moves the hips in preparation for the birth, and wakens up the spine.

6. BADDHA KONASANA

COBBLER POSE

Continuing from Bharadvajasana, bring the soles of your feet together a comfortable distance away from your hips (lefthand picture). If there is any strain on your hips or knees then take your feet further away from you. To wake up your spine, spiral your whole spine round to the right from the base, so that you face around over your right knee. Take your right fingertips onto the ground to the right. Repeat to the left (middle picture), then sit lengthened up through the spine. If the spine can stay

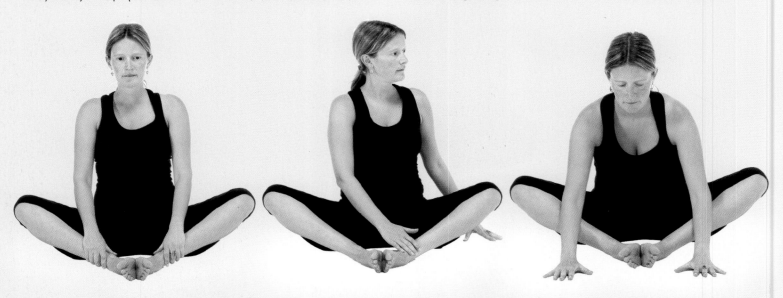

lengthened, take the fingers forward to bring the spine forward and up (righthand picture, previous page). If your back is at all under strain, then sit with your back against the wall and a blanket comfortably wedged just above your sacrum, as in the

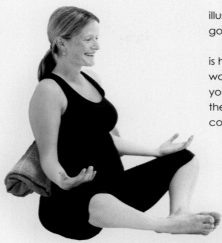

illustration on this page. This is a good posture for meditation.

NB: Yoga teachers: this pose is helpful if you have pregnant women in a general class. Let your pregnant students sit against the wall for as long as they are comfortable, with a blanket rolled

and wedged at the level of the top of the sacrum and lumbar spine, while you are doing another pose, maybe a twist that your pregnant students shouldn't do, with the rest of the class.

> YOGA IS THE SETTLING OF THE MIND
> INTO SILENCE.
> WHEN THE MIND HAS SETTLED,
> WE ARE ESTABLISHED IN OUR
> ESSENTIAL NATURE, WHICH IS
> UNBOUNDED CONSCIOUSNESS.
> OUR ESSENTIAL NATURE IS USUALLY
> OVERSHADOWED BY THE ACTIVITY
> OF THE MIND.
> THE YOGA SUTRAS OF PATANJALI,
> TRANSLATED BY ALISTAIR SHEARER

7. DANDASANA
STAFF POSE

Points to watch: *make sure that the thigh bones are relaxed back into hips to move spine upwards and forwards. The fingers should be spreading down into the ground and the feet active and alive*

Points to watch: *have hips just the right distance from the wall so that the thighs release out of the hip joint. If you are too close to the wall it will restrict the baby*

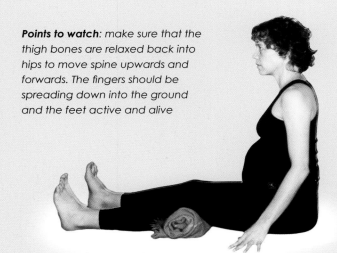

From *Baddha konasana,* Cobbler pose, on the previous pages, stretch your legs straight out in front of you. If this causes you any strain in your back, you can put a folded blanket underneath your knees so they are not pushed down, or lie with your legs up the wall in *Urdhva dandasana* – the same pose but upside down.

Spread your fingertips down, or onto the chair in front of you, to lengthen your arms and spine up. Spread into your heels.

8. PARSVATASANA
CROSS-LEGGED MOUNTAIN POSE

Points to watch: *extend the spine forward and upward, the brow resting down. Keep the feet active and spreading into the heels*

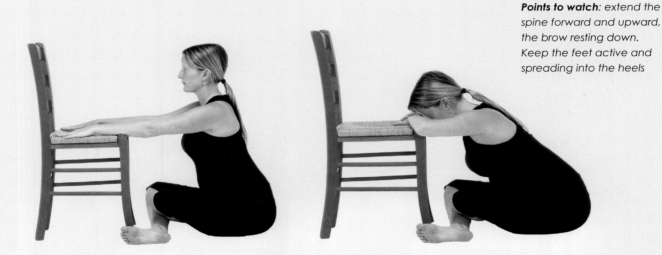

From *Dandasana*, Staff pose, cross your legs, extending into your heels. Stretch your spine upwards by placing your hands on a chair as shown. Spread into your heels, hands and shoulders to let the spine lengthen up through the shoulderblades.

Rest your arms and brow onto the chair in front of you. Stay there for at least a minute and up to four, breathing gently into your back ribs. Then change the cross of your legs and repeat.

This posture relaxes the head and brain, and relieves headaches, high blood-pressure, backache and strain in the hips. It also restores energy.

9. Paschimottanasana
SITTING FORWARD BEND

Stretching your legs out underneath the chair in front of you, place your hands around the back and ease it away from you until your spine feels extended forward and up, and then spread your hands down to increase the lengthening of your spine up, then rest forward with your brow on the chair for one to four minutes.

This posture calms the mind, especially when the head is rested down, and lengthens the spine out of the hips.

All the last three postures wake up the whole spinal column, open the hip joints ready for childbirth, relax the head, and reduce blood-pressure and headaches.

Points to watch: *in both positions, keep the heels and feet spreading; lengthen the legs back from the heels to move the spine out of the hips*

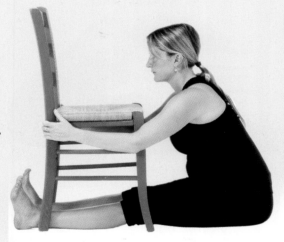 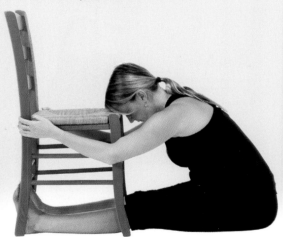

10. SETU BANDHA SARVANGASANA
BRIDGE POSE

Now lie down on your back with knees bent and feet flat down, arms rested out to the side (as below). Spread down through your heels and up through your calves to take knees down and away so that the hips lift (do not push the hips up, let the legs do the work!). Move the spine towards your head, so that there is a two-way extension (right). You can then put support under your sacrum as shown (bottom right), so that you can rest there for a few minutes. Or you can come down and go again as each time you are able bring more awareness more down through your feet.

Do not do this posture if there is any strain in your head, neck or across your tummy.

It eases the spine out and back after carrying extra weight, moves the hips and relieves heartburn and helps any strain in the digestion.

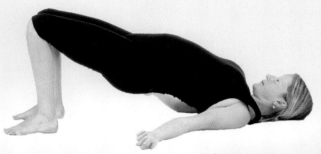

Points to watch: keep the heels firmly down, and bring the shinbones straight up out of the ankle bones

Points to watch: thighbones should be resting into the hip joint; extend the spine, towards the head

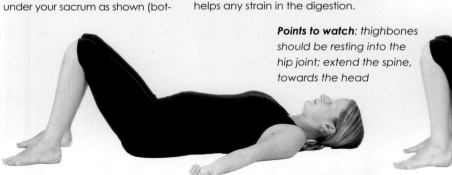

11. SAVASANA
RELAXATION

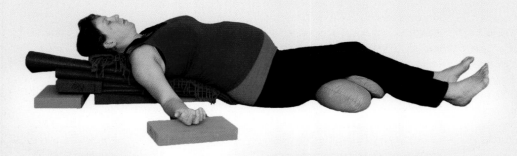

Lie down on your back with plenty of support for the upper back – and for the hands as well, if needed. If this is not comfortable, roll onto your side and rest there, with a blanket or block wedged into the back for support.

Savasana is translated as Corpse pose. However, that word is not intended literally, neither do you go to sleep in it, although you may have a necessary phase of doing that if you have a deficit of sleep! Eventually, you need to remain awake and alert for it, the body not flopped, yet relaxed.

An Indian teacher I went to once described it as 'the balance between the Cow dung pose and the Stick pose'! So the mind and eyes are relaxed down towards the body, aware of your breathing, and aware of the points of contact with the earth underneath you. Thus your whole body rests back and is supported by mother earth. In turn, this will support you in your new, most vital role of mother.

12. Nadi Sodhana in Savasana
ALTERNATE NOSTRIL BREATHING IN RELAXATION AND IN SITTING

Nadi sodhana literally means cleansing of the nadiis or energy channels, but it is generally called alternate nostril breathing as this is how you cleanse the channels.

Let your breath gently come and go, focusing on your back body, especially your ribs. When you are ready, bring your awareness to your left side, to let your breath come more through that side – right from the pelvic floor – into your left lungs and your left nostril. Then exhale through your left side.

You may feel you want to open your fingers or toes. This does help the opening of the lungs and nostril tremendously as you are engaging a mudra or gesture that affects the whole body. After a few breaths, take an easy breath, then transfer your awareness to the other side and repeat.

Do not rush the moment of moving onto this stage – you may feel to stay with the first section for a while of practice – but if and when you feel ready let your breath come in through the left side to the top of the inhalation and out through the right side, then breath in through the right side and out through the left side.

Continue this movement of your breath from side to side. Finish on the left side where you started, then let the breath come in through both sides, feeling if it is so much easier to breathe fully now. When you are ready to get up, roll over onto your left side, rest there for a few moments and gently come up from your side to sitting, spending a moment or two or longer communicating with your baby, feeling any awareness you might have, for the practice of yoga opens up our awareness to our body and what is going on there. You can sit now for *Nadi sodhana* using the lotus mudra to help the opening of your body to your breath, as shown in the pictures.

Close your fingers as shown

Points to watch: *start with fingers closed like a flower in bud. Opening the fingers on one side as you inhale emphasizes the breathe coming in through the nostril on that side*

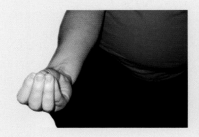 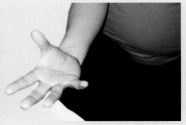

NADHI SODHANA, SEATED IN A CROSS-LEGGED POSTURE USING THE PADMA (LOTUS) MUDRA

on the previous page, all fingers touching the thumb as a lotus or tulip. Then as your breath comes in, open the fingers on your left hand, like a lotus opening out. As you reach the top of the inhalation, close the left fingers opening the right fingers. Do this as long as your awareness can stay with it. Then gently breathe through both nostrils, feeling the clearing effect of Nadi sodhana.

This breathing practice balances the two sides of your body, relieves headaches, and reduces high blood-pressure, and cleanses and calms the whole system.

There is a section on chanting, mudras, breathing and meditation in the next chapter, on labour, which can be practised any time, to prepare you and for you to be able to practise them in labour.

To relax is not to collapse, but simply to undo tension. This tension has been accumulated in the body and in the mind by years of forceful education. Tension is the result of will, effort and prejudice. We have been trained, during the first part of our lives to struggle to achieve. Now we can to work in the opposite direction, by letting go, giving place to a different action, an 'undoing action'. This will stop the habitual process of doing which has become mechanical.

The body itself is healthy, but it has been ruined by all sorts of negative, destructive, guilt feelings. If one can avoid going in this negative direction, a positive attitude will take over and the body will then be able to start its recuperative function, its natural way of existing.

There is nothing to be done.

It is not a state of passivity but on the contrary, of watchful alertness. It is perhaps the most 'active' of our attitudes, going 'with' and not 'against' our body and feelings.

Vanda Scaravelli, AWAKENING THE SPINE

Midwifery Notes
with Helpful Postures

PREGNANCY-INDUCED HYPERTENSION

Otherwise known as pre-eclampsia, this is a condition that occurs in later pregnancy and is associated with a rise in the diastolic blood-pressure, protein present in the urine (proteinuria) and oedema. Other symptoms include epigastric pain, headaches and blurred vision.

The cause is largely unknown but recent studies suggest that a likely cause is abnormal implantation of the placenta which results in decreased placental perfusion which leads to lack of oxygen to the placenta so causing it to release chemicals which damage the body organs leading to the symptoms of raised blood-pressure, proteinuria and oedema.

This is a life-threatening condition for the mother and the baby if it is not controlled, as ultimately the mother may have an eclamptic fit. Thus the control of the condition is desirable as early delivery of the foetus is the only other way to remedy the problem.

Yoga postures
All Sitting forward bends using a chair to rest head on for two to four minutes each time, will reduce blood-pressure. Follow with Relaxation with good support for the upper back, or lying on the left side if more comfortable, breathing gently into the back ribs. See the postures earlier in this chapter, *Janu sirsasana* (p. 86), *Parsvatasana* (p. 91) and *Paschimottanasana* (p. 92).

DIGESTIVE SYSTEM

As the end of the pregnancy approaches, the stomach attains a vertical position rather than a horizontal one which results in greater intergastric pressure and greater oesophageal reflux and heartburn. As the uterus is very large at this point, the stomach is also displaced upwards and the resulting gastric symptoms are very difficult to treat. Constipation and haemorrhoids are also a difficult and uncomfortable problem, due to the effects of raised levels of progesterone at this stage leading to longer transit time and increased colonic water absorption. Oral iron preparations contribute to the problem.

Appetite is greatly affected because of the large uterus displacing the stomach and obstructing it so decreasing its capacity, so women have to eat a little and often.

Yoga postures
Bharadvajasana (Mermaid pose, p. 87), using a wall to the side or chair in front to put hand on. *Dandasana* (Staff pose, p. 90), using a support under the knees and a belt or chair to stretch the spine up,

Janu sirsasana (p. 86) – using a chair if needed. *Baddha konasana* (p. 88), *Adho mukha svanasana* (p. 67), *Viparita karani* (p. 68), supported *Halasana* (Plough pose, p. 69), making sure there is no strain in the face.

CARDIOVASCULAR SYSTEM

The heart rate in the third trimester will increase and become ten to fifteen beats a minute faster than in the first trimester. The uterus at this late stage of pregnancy receives seventeen percent of the cardiac output, the breasts two percent, while in the other organs the output remains much the same throughout the pregnancy. Supine hypotension is an increasing problem in the last trimester and can manifest in bradycardia (slow heart rate) dizziness, light-headedness and nausea. Again, lying on the left side results in cardiac output being restored and these symptoms dissipating.

Yoga postures
Anapanasati (calming breathing, p. 48), in all postures and all activities. *Supta virasana* (p. 82), *Malasana* (p. 65) – both of these should be well supported.

Savasana and meditation (p. 94), chanting OM, *Hridaya mudra* (Heart gesture, see photo below).

MUSCULOSKELETAL SYSTEM

Oestrogen, progesterone and relaxin continue to influence the joints, connective tissue and ligaments at this stage of pregnancy, often resulting in marked lordosis (the spine bends backwards and the shoulder girdle slumps to maintain the woman's centre of gravity over her feet).

This results in low back pain and the stretching of the abdominal muscles which in turn lose tone; it also contributes to backache. The *rectus abdominis* muscle (muscle on the anterior wall of the stomach stretching from the ribs to the *symphisis pubis*) can divide in the late stage of pregnancy, and after delivery can be palpated

up to 4 cm apart and sometimes take up to six months to repair. Oestrogen and progesterone continue to affect the pelvic ligaments and joints in preparation for the foetal passage.

Cramp is another uncomfortable side effect of late pregnancy, with the cause largely unknown and the only real remedy, apparently, leg extension and local massage.

Yoga postures
Pindasana (Child pose, pp. 29, 83), Dog (p. 67), *Dandasana* (Staff) and *Urdhva dandasana* (with legs up the wall) (p. 90), *Viparita karani* (Reversing attitude pose, p. 68) and Wide-angle posture (*Upavistha konasana*, p. 84).

URINARY SYSTEM

The most common problem in late pregnancy is frequency of micturition (passing urine) and nocturia (passing urine at night). This is due to the increased blood volume which in turn results in increased production of urine and also the bladder has a reduced capacity due to the very large uterus so can only hold small amounts of urine.

Yoga postures
All the poses that are given for the second and third trimesters.

BREATHING

Respiration is affected by stress and one of the easiest ways of assisting relaxation is by becoming aware of your breath, which will then bring it to its natural length and rhythm. This will take several minutes of lying down in relaxation with your eyes relaxed and as though looking downwards towards the rest of your body. Slow, deep inhalation followed by complete exhalation will help to relax the mother and therefore the foetus too. Natural, rhythmic breathing is the most beneficial and if this skill is taught late on in pregnancy it can be most useful, if not essential, to help cope with early labour and sometimes the more advanced stages of labour.

Very slow deep breathing can cause hyperventilation which can lead to light-headedness and tingling in the fingers. This can be remedied by cupping the hands over the mouth and re-breathing your own carbon dioxide, therefore rebalancing the oxygen/carbon dioxide levels. Shallow breathing or panting is a very useful technique to learn for the acute phases in labour but should only be practised intermittently as it will cause hypoventilation (abnormally slow breathing) and subsequent oxygen deprivation.

So the emphasis should be placed on easy, rhythmic breathing which aids relaxation of the mother and is also a quick way to re-energize.

Yoga postures
Anapanasati (calming breathing, p. 48) emphasizing spreading into the back ribs and ladder breath on exhalation. This can be practised in *Supta virasana* (Extending-the-spine Hero pose, p. 82), *Savasana* (relaxation or sitting in meditation, p. 94).

WHEN WE STAND, WE CREATE A CHANNEL FROM EARTH TO HEAVEN. ENERGY FLOWS AND CREATES US AND CONTINUES THAT PROCESS EVERY SECOND. THAT'S WHY ALL OUR CELLS GET RENEWED.

NOW, IF YOU WATCH A BONE, THE LONG ONES IN THE LEG, YOU WILL NOTICE THAT THEY DON'T DIFFER MUCH FROM BAMBOO. THEY ARE HOLLOW. WHAT LIVES INSIDE THAT SPACE? BONE MARROW, WHERE RED BLOOD CELLS ARE CREATED.

LIFE-FORCE STREAMS THROUGH THESE CHANNELS. FROM THE FOOT ARCHES IT FLOWS THROUGH THESE CHANNELS, UP AND OUT TO THE SKY. ONCE YOU ARE AWARE OF THIS, YOU CAN DROP YOUR 'HARD' WORK AND ENJOY A DEEP AWARENESS OF BEING A STREAMING BEING, CARRIED AND BEING TAKEN CARE OF BY MOTHER NATURE.

VICTOR VAN KOOTEN, FROM INSIDE OUT

GOING OVERDUE

Unlike animals, humans do not have an exact gestation time and it can be anything from thirty-seven weeks to forty-two weeks. It is said to be around two hundred and eighty days, give or take ten. There are several variables too. The length of a woman's cycle, her confidence as to the date of her last menstrual period and if she has recently been on the Pill. Ultrasound is used to give an estimate of the due date and can be accurate to within five days. And then it is important to remember that we are not all the same size and this applies to the foetus too! The problem with going overdue is that the placenta has a lifespan of approximately forty-two weeks, after which it begins to deteriorate thereby affecting the oxygen and the nutrients getting to the foetus.

Only one percent of babies are born on their due date. Some are born before but most (particularly in a first pregnancy) are born up to two weeks after 'the date' the woman has been given. In my experience if women are prepared for this outcome they can prepare mentally for it. As yet no-one really knows how labour starts, whether it is foetally or maternally led, but it is generally accepted that the cervix 'ripens' (becomes softer and more compliant) and the increasing pressure of the foetal head on the cervix aids the commencement of labour. So the 'old-fashioned' methods of bringing labour on can have a real effect. The long walks, the bumpy car ride, the castor oil (!) and, of course, sex can all bring on labour—intercourse because there are prostaglandins in the sperm which 'mimic' the natural chemicals produced as increasing pressure is exerted on the cervix by the foetal head. Although this is probably 'too much information' as they say, rear entry is best for the deepest penetration!!

YOGA

The date given you is not always exact: it cannot be for humans as it varies and you yourself sometimes have more of a sense than anyone of when the baby is ready, as it is the baby's system that initiates labour. Sally gives several ways of instigating labour.

I have also found the practice programme that follows has always worked unless a Caesarean section, planned or emergency, is required or the baby is 'in breech' – i.e., the baby is turned around so that the feet or bottom will come out first.

Only use the programme on the next page when you are overdue your given date, and in conjunction with a teacher who has access to the following note.

NOTE TO YOGA TEACHERS

Only give this set of suggestions if your student is overdue and only when they have gone past their due date and teach them solely to the overdue mother, as they are yoga postures that you wouldn't normally do at this stage. You will need the help of at least one other teacher or student teacher.

Please do not do this if you are not happy to do so. My experience is that it works within twenty-four hours and that it is preferable to being induced.

Work in the following order:

a) Walking into the standing postures, moving quite fast and taking arms up overhead (for about twenty minutes). If you can do this outside, it is even better.

b) Follow this with ten minutes of *Baddha Konasana* against a wall.

c) If you feel confident, and are able to provide two helpers who also feel happy to help you, then continue with *Salamba Sirsasana* (supported Headstand, not shown in this book) between two chairs, making sure that the face is not going red or looking strained. You could move your pupil into preparation for

Headstand if they are used to doing it, or halfway with the shoulders supported on the chairs and the legs slightly elevated on a low stool. Make sure you only do this with practised yoga students, and that you have someone there to help you, preferably two people – one either side – otherwise leave it out.

d) Lying with legs up the wall.

e) Shoulderstand from the wall, as shown below (more detail on pp. 69–70).

If you feel unsure at all about doing this routine but would like advice or the possibility of a one-to-one, please contact The Inner Yoga Trust.

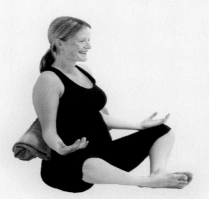

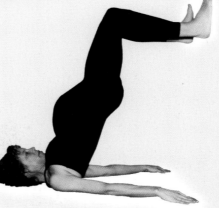

THOUGH NOT YET BORN, I HAVE THE BABY WITH ME. AT NIGHT, BEFORE I TRY TO SLEEP, I BREATHE IN AND DOWN, IMAGINE MYSELF SINKING THROUGH MY BODY TO REACH THE LIFE INSIDE. I SEE THE GOLDEN BABY THROUGH THE DARKNESS, MOVE CLOSER TO CHALICE THE CHILD IN MY ARMS, POURING MY LIFEBLOOD INTO AND THROUGH THE LIGHT. I THINK: 'IF, BY SOME DARK CHANCE, WE NEVER GET TO MEET, IF I NEVER GET TO HEAR YOUR VOICE OR YOU NEVER SEE ME SMILE, KNOW THIS: YOUR MOTHER LOVED YOU'.

JUDITH O'REILLY, WIFE IN THE NORTH

5. Labour and Childbirth and the Month Before

AS WE GET nearer our due date, a combination of anticipation, fear and excitement come in; a longing to see this baby we have carried for nine months. Inevitably, there is some fear and trepidation around the whole process of labour and birth as we never know how that is going to proceed. We often have plans, things we definitely want to happen and things we don't. It can all turn out so differently, in fact; there is such a huge range of eventualities!

If we have established a regular practice of yoga and meditation, then we will be able to go with whatever is happening – and needs to happen – far more readily and easily, trusting those around us are doing the best for us and the baby. Through our regular practice we will also be much more in control of our own body and mind and able to relax and go with what is needed.

If you can read and practise what is given in this chapter for the month before you are due, you will be able to put it into practice as soon as your labour commences. Remember that the breathing, chanting and mudras can be practised in any position, anywhere – a minute's practice or opening of awareness will make a difference to how you are throughout your labour and childbirth. I have even known women who have had to get onto all fours in the back of a car on the way to the hospital, as they found it the most comfortable position to be in. So maybe the postures can be done anywhere, too!

I can remember walking around the field next to the hospital after I had been admitted. I had not gone into labour, so after several hours I felt as though I was going to be nine months' pregnant for the rest of my life – so I breathed gently, pausing on the exhalation. I did a gentle *Viloma* breath in rhythm with my walking pace and that calmed me down.

I felt then I just needed patience and trust in those around me, the ability to go with the outcome whatever it was, as I did know at that stage that the baby's heart was irregular, but did not know how that would be managed. The obstetrician continually monitored the baby's heartbeat, but did not give me any information other than that he was not happy about it. Curiously, he reminded me of my first yoga teacher, Kofi Busia. Kofi, it seemed to me, was the teacher who had initated me into my life path – with no particular ceremony, but that was how it felt. The obstetrician was possibly from Ghana, with an impeccable Oxford accent, just like Kofi.

ANATOMY OF BIRTH

THE PELVIS

The pelvis is made of four different types of bones:
- two innominate bones (hip bones)
- one sacrum
- one coccyx

Each innominate bone is made up of three bones which have fused together. These are the ilium or ileum (the large flared-out section), the ischium (the thick lower part) and the pubic bone which forms the anterior part.

The ischium has a large prominence, the ischial tuberosity, and it is on this the body rests when sitting. Just up from there is the ischial spine which protrudes into the pelvic space. When the woman is in labour it is here that the descent of the foetal head is measured and progress is assessed.

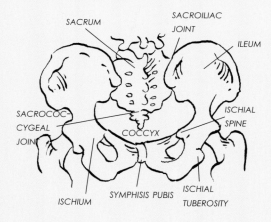

BONE STRUCTURE IN THE PELVIC REGION, VIEWED FROM THE FRONT OF THE BODY

The sacrum consists of five fused vertebrae. The anterior (forward) surface is referred to as the hollow of the sacrum.

The coccyx consists of four fused vertebrae and is our 'tail'. During the last stage of labour this will bend backwards to allow the foetus to pass through.

THE PELVIC JOINTS AND LIGAMENTS

There are four pelvic joints:
- one *symphisis pubis*
- two sacroiliac joints
- one sacrococcygeal joint

The *symphisis pubis* is the joint where the two pubic bones meet. It is cushioned by a pad of cartilage and held together by the interpubic ligaments.

The two sacroiliac joints are the strongest in the body, as they join the sacrum to the ilium and thus connect the spine to the pelvis. The sacroiliac ligaments connect the sacrum to the ilium.

The sacrococcygeal joint is between the sacrum and the coccyx and is held together by the sacrococcygeal ligaments.

During pregnancy the ligaments soften under the influence of progesterone and relaxin and this causes the pelvis to have some flexibility to move and widen to allow the passage of the foetus through in labour. In some women the symphisis pubis may separate slightly causing pain on walking. Lower backache is common too as the sacroiliac joints come under the influence of these pregnancy hormones as well.

THE FOETUS

The parietal bones are the large bones which lay either side of the foetal skull and the parietal eminence is the prominent are on this bone. The bi-parietal diameter is the measured distance between the parietal eminences of the foetal skull.

The frontal bones lie at the front of the foetal skull and the occipital bone at the back. The occiput is the prominent area on the occipital bone.

The posterior fontanelle is the membrane space bordered by the occiput and the parietal bones and the anterior fontanelle is the membranous space bordered by the frontal bones and the parietal bones.

– Presentation: this is the part of the foetus lying in the lower uterine segment over the cervical os. In normal labour this is the head and the presentation is said to be 'cephalic'.

– Position: the relationship of the presenting part to six points on the pelvis. In normal labour this is the relationship of the occiput of the foetal skull to the left or right anterior, lateral or posterior aspect of the pelvis – most usually, left occipito anterior.

– Foetal skull: this contains the very delicate brain and is large in comparison with the foetal body and the maternal pelvis. The head is the most difficult part to be born and the part over which most care must be taken. At the time of birth the bones of the foetal skull have not completely ossified and are separate which allows them to override one another during the passage through the pelvis and therefore successfully negotiate the bony birth canal.

The pelvis is the bony canal through which the foetus must pass during birth. It consists of a brim, a cavity and an outlet. With knowledge of the presentation, position and flexion of the foetus and the strength and length of contractions it is possible to anticipate the descent of the foetal skull through the pelvis and, therefore, along with other observations of the mother and the foetus, establish whether normal labour is in progress and, if not, take correct action.

The pelvic brim is the narrowest part of the pelvis and the bi-parietal diameter of the foetal skull is the widest part. So when the widest part of the foetal skull passes through the brim of the pelvis, engagement of the foetal skull is said to have taken place. This is significant because, generally speaking, what goes in will come out!!! In a primigravid (first-time mum) this is expected to happen around thirty-six to thirty-seven weeks pregnant. However in a multigravida (second and subsequent pregnancies) this sometimes does not happen until labour is established. This does not usually cause concern as she has already 'proven' her pelvis by already having given birth to a full-term infant.

THE PELVIC FLOOR

This is the double layer of muscle lying over the pelvic outlet. The most important of these is the strong hammock-like muscle through which passes the urethra (tube from the bladder to the outside of the body), the vagina and the anal canal. Obviously these muscles are under enormous strain in late pregnancy, and during labour they relax to allow the passive movement of the foetus through the birth canal. It is generally in the postnatal period that we need to focus attention on these muscles and there is argument as to whether active perineal exercise aids healing or a more passive, gentle approach has greater longterm

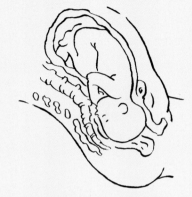

RELATIONSHIP OF THE BABY TO THE SPINE IN A WOMAN READY TO GIVE BIRTH (RESTING BACK)

effect. Also, moderate strengthening exercises and direct massage in the antenatal period is thought to have some beneficial effect.

THE UTERUS

By the end of pregnancy the uterus has formed into the upper uterine segment and the lower uterine segment. The upper segment forms the majority of the uterus and is thick and muscular. The lower uterine segment is thinner muscle and is mainly concerned with distension and dilation of the cervix. During labour the upper segment contracts and retracts pulling on the lower uterine segment which distends and dilates.

CERVICAL EFFACEMENT

During the latter part of pregnancy the cervix gradually merges into the lower uterine segment and becomes part of it, so there is no perceptible canal between the internal and the external cervical os. This is often accompanied by 'Braxton Hicks' contractions which are preparatory contractions often mistaken for the 'real' thing, the main difference being that the periods of Braxton Hicks are spasmodic, irregular and sometimes not all that painful and diminish. Also, there is no dilation of the cervix.

LABOUR

THE ONSET OF NORMAL LABOUR

Labour is divided into three stages. The first stage of labour is from the onset of regular uterine contractions to the full dilation of the cervix to ten centimetres. The second stage of labour is from full dilation to the birth of the baby and the third stage of labour is from the birth of the baby until the placenta and membranes have been fully expelled and any bleeding controlled. In a primigravid woman (one pregnant for the first time) the first stage of labour is on average twelve to fourteen hours long and in a multigravid woman about six to ten hours.

It is thought that labour starts as a result of the pressure of the foetal head on the cervix causing an increase in the secretion of oestrogen which, in turn, causes the muscle fibres of the upper uterine segment to contract and retract.

Generally speaking, labour establishes slowly, aptly named the latent phase, when there is less uterine activity and slow dilation of the cervix. As contractions become longer, stronger and more intense the cervix dilates more rapidly and this is called the active phase of labour. There is often a phase of labour called transition, or sometimes a 'state of change', which occurs at the end of the first stage of labour and before the second. Often characterized by very strong and long, painful, frequently unbearable contractions followed by a long, much needed period of rest. This is the time when some women think that death would be preferable!

NORMAL MECHANISM OF LABOUR

The foetal head is well flexed i.e. the chin well tucked into the chest and enters the pelvis in a left occipital anterior position, i.e., with the occiput pointing towards the left anterior pubic bone. As labour progresses, the occiput is pushed downwards onto the pelvic floor and the resistance of this muscle brings about rotation of the foetal head into the anterior posterior position in preparation for birth.

All through this part of labour, the head is negotiating its way through the largest diameters of the pelvic brim, cavity and outlet. Once the head is born the shoulders (usually smaller in diameter than the head) follow with a similar twist in the pelvis, and the anterior shoulder now lies in the anterior posterior position, the head 'restitutes' to line up with the shoulders and the occiput now lies laterally.

METHODS FOR DEALING WITH PAIN

Every woman's perception of pain is different and each person has their own individual way of dealing with it. There are the orthodox methods available (TENS, entonox, pethidine and epidural). Water labour and birth are becoming increasingly available. All of these have advantages and disadvantages.

There is no doubt that breathing techniques are very useful, and for some women are all they use throughout. It would seem beneficial to the woman to remain centred within herself, responding to her body's own needs and staying in touch with the natural progress of labour. Fear and anxiety raise the levels of adrenaline in the bloodstream and the woman can easily feel out of control and very frightened. In my experience, it is important to reassure and encourage her that the sensations she is experiencing are all normal and that labour is progressing along its natural pathway.

The ambience of the setting is important as it is implicit trust between her and her birth supporters. If it is her second or subsequent child, then the woman will need to know her other children are being well cared for.

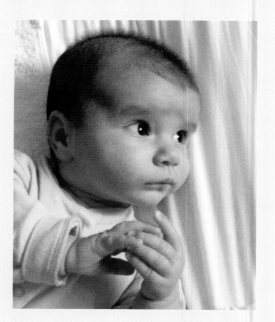

POSITIONS TO ENCOURAGE THE FOETUS INTO THE OPTIMAL POSITION FOR BIRTH

While some women will have made a birth plan and have in their mind an 'ideal outcome', I have found that a real sense of openmindedness is vital to avoid the 'hope/disillusionment' cycle, and, also, the deep seated sense of failure some women feel if they have not given birth in their (or anyone else's) pre-chosen way.

Birth itself is a gift and to be able to give life is a gift and sometimes things don't always go to plan. It is therefore wise for neither the mother nor her yoga teacher to become fixed on any outcome apart from healthy mother and baby! Midwives are well trained professionals who want the best for mum and babe and, sometimes, with all their knowledge and experience they make decisions which are in everyone's best interests but don't necessarily follow the prescribed 'plan'.

SECOND STAGE OF LABOUR

Uterine contractions are strong, expulsive and aid the descent of the head through the birth canal. Gravity can be a great assistant at this time as a woman uses strength she often never knew she had to push the baby out. As the head 'crowns' (the widest biparietal diameter distends the vulva and no longer recedes between contractions) the utmost care and control needs to be exercised by mum and midwife at this point to aid maximum perineal stretching and safe, gentle delivery of the head. Panting breathing 'like a dog' is often recommended which promotes slow, gradual delivery of the head and enables the mother to remain fully in control. After delivery of the head, rotation of the shoulders takes place and restitution of the head and, generally, with the next contraction the body is born.

THIRD STAGE OF LABOUR

The unique characteristic of uterine muscle lies in its ability to retract. After expulsion of the foetus, the uterus gets smaller quite quickly and the placental site diminishes in size. As this occurs, the placenta becomes compressed and detaches itself from the uterine wall. Separation is further aided by the formation of a retroplacental clot which exerts further pressure on the placenta resulting in separation. While gravity can help the separation and delivery of the placenta and membranes, very often the new parents are exhausted and exhilarated and find sitting or lying down cradling the newborn the most comfortable way to welcome the new life into the world.

POSTURES DURING LABOUR

The postures, breathing, chanting and mudras given here, as was said in the last chapter, can be practised at any time in pregnancy to prepare for this momentous and important time in your life. On the IYT pregnancy module we use a chart from The National Childbirth Trust (see p. 156); the postures here help the positions given on that sheet.

You will need a large gymnastic ball (for suppliers see p. 156). This can be used instead of a chair, in yoga poses; a firmly pumped-up ball is much better on the spine than a chair as there is some give in the ball which enables the pelvic floor to work more efficiently for breathing and for moving the spine. Make sure in the days of prepara-tion that it's kept firmly pumped up and get used to using it.

In the first stage of labour (see Sally's notes, p. 107), sit on the ball

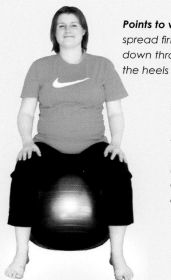

Points to watch: *spread firmly down through the heels*

and, with your feet set wide apart and firmly on the ground, spread back and down into your heels, so that you can bounce gently up

Points to watch: *shoulders need to be relaxed and the spine forward and up, while the knees remain over the ankles.*

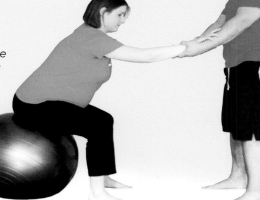

and down from the base of your spine. This releases and moves the spine all the way up to the top of your neck. This will   be

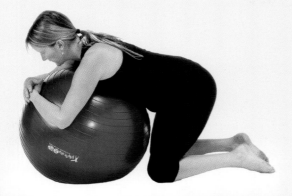

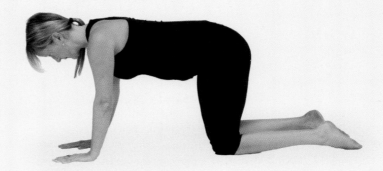

very soothing during contractions.

You birthing partner can hold your wrists in front of you and gently extend your whole spine forwards, which opens the base area, encouraging the baby down (see opposite). You can swing your arms from side to side so that the spine gently twists on its axis.

When that's enough come forward onto your knees and bring the ball around in front of you, so you can rest your upper body forward and down onto the ball. This is Child pose, modified for pregnancy and childbirth.

Relax here as long as comfortable during contractions. When it's

enough, tuck your toes under and roll back onto you feet into a squat (photo p. 65), you can have help in front as shown, or have the wall behind you (photo p. 66). Again, it is helpful to have a bounce and a chant there and have that feeling of going with the contractions.

Then come forward onto your

knees and hands, on all fours. This is a very comfortable position for the first and second stage of labour and one that you can be in for a time, as that position of the spine parallel to the ground gives a good posture for the baby to move down the birth canal and is a good place to do the chants given next.

MAKING SOUNDS

Chanting, singing, making birthing sounds, even swearing, are all ways of expression that women have found themselves spontaneously doing during labour – probably since the beginning of humankind and animal kind. (Animals make wonderful noises at this time.)

So this may be completely spontaneou,s or you may feel you want to use these chants to start with and beforehand to get your voice and awareness ready so there is no self-consciousness.

In her notes for the second stage of labour, Sally says that panting like a dog is recommended. This has some similarities to the *Kapalabhati* breath given next.

PRANAYAMA (KAPALABHATI BREATH)

As I described at the end of Chapter 3 (p. 72), start by gently extending the exhalation for a few breaths, bringing in the pauses on the exhalation as described under *Viloma*, the ladder breath.

Kapalabhati means 'shining skull breath' or 'that which brings lightness to the skull'. It's also called dragon breath.

For the *Kapalabhati* breath,

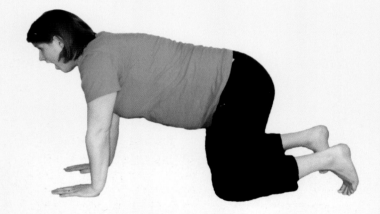

gently inhale, and on the exhalation breathe out in a series of little snorts, as you might do after running – indeed you may feel as though you have been running during labour! This exhalation would help you to go with the contractions.

Breathe in easily, to repeat the little snorts on the next exhalation. You will find that the breath comes in more easily after a few *Kapalabhati* exhalations. When it's enough, take a gentle inhalation then feel a long, smooth exhalation naturally comes. Then do another round of five to ten breaths. Rest when the contractions stop for a while.

SOUNDING OR CHANTING

The sound OM, in its three phases expressed as the sounds A-U-M, is described in yoga as the sound that created the Universe. This is in fact just what you are doing in giving birth to your child: you are providing form for the Universal. So for this sound to be chanted loud and clear is very appropriate at all stages of labour.

You need to open your mouth really wide for the A (ah) to come out strongly. I was taught to put three fingers side by side in my mouth to get the width needed. Then bring your lips in, but still a little open for the U (oo), closing your lips for the M (mm). This can be over three breaths if you like, gradually going into one breath. The sound may change as you progress with it. For instance, it may become I AM, a strong statement affirming who you are.

This sounding brings you into your

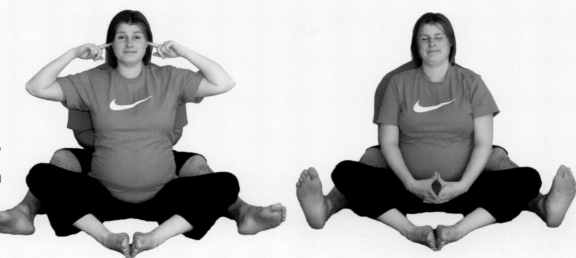

full power, ready to expel the baby.

This sound is very appropriate for the more active time of labour, when the contractions are strong and coming fast. When there is a pause you may like to do the *Bhramari* or Bee breath.

You can do your chanting with your partner behind you to support you, as shown in the photos.

BHRAMARI OR BEE BREATH

Take an easy inhalation, and then on the exhalation, with your mouth closed, make a sound just like a bee humming, shown here (left) with an index finger in each ear to start with as you can then hear the sound very strongly and clearly. The sound is rather like OM. This breath

is very calming at this stage.

During this *Bhramari* breath you can put your fingers in the *Yoni* mudra shown right, with the index fingers and the thumbs touching, the other fingers linked. *Yoni* is the Sanskrit word used to describe the vaginal opening at the base, so you are encouraging this opening by using this *hasta mudra* or hand gesture.

ABNORMAL LABOUR AND BIRTH

This is what all women fear, and so it needs to be addressed as Sally has below. I wanted to give my own personal experience of this first.

I was aware during my one pregnancy of some fear about the actual process of labour and childbirth and very much used my yoga practice in all its aspects of the Eight Limbs of yoga.

There felt, being a yoga teacher, to be from myself, as well as others, some pressure to have the ideal birth. Sally was so helpful in this as my independent midwife.

So when she detected a few days before the birth that the foetal heartbeat was not clear, I did not know what to expect but trusted Sally and the hospital to know what to do.

My waters broke at 1 a.m. I did not want to ring Sally then as I knew she had attended a long delivery the day before, and so I meditated for nearly six hours, until 7 a.m. This was a glorious time of expectation, fear, excitement and change. I have never meditated for so long before or since, but I know that it is regular practice for Buddhist monks and nuns on moon nights (full, new and half moons).

It stood me in good stead for all that happened during the birth – and right up to now, really, when my daughter has at last come through very difficult teenage years.

After my waters breaking, nothing happened for the next twenty-four hours except a lot of monitoring of Beth's heartbeat. I was afraid they would want to induce her, which did not intuitively feel right to me. Then suddenly at 2 a.m the following morning (a very long twenty-five hours), the Consultant obstetrician announced he wanted to perform a Caesarean section. This was a shock to my mind, as I had not considered it at all. Yet I was aware that my whole body, and perhaps the baby too, went into relief and relaxed.

I give this personal example, as Sally says we get attached to a particular outcome but we need to go with whatever *is* and trust. The practice of yoga greatly enables this process of going with and trusting the universe. I believe this trust may actually affect the outcome. In this case when the consultant came the next day, he said he was surprised to find that the baby was quite all right. I thank Sally every day for the life of my daughter, as her vigilance beforehand made the hospital take special care.

MIDWIFERY NOTES

Sally aptly divided her notes here under three headings:
Powers!!
Passages!!
Passengers!!

Powers

The powers in normal labour are the parts of the anatomy that 'power' the foetus down towards and through the birth canal. Broadly speaking, these are the muscles of the uterus and the overall strength of the woman. If, for some reason, one or other of these fails then the 'powers' are compromised and the labour will deviate from 'normal'. Also, if the body fails to commence labour between the thirty-seventh week of pregnancy and the forty-second week then she will need help and the labour is said to be 'abnormal'.

The most common reason for the powers to fail is that the woman has a very prolonged labour and becomes totally exhausted. This, contributed to by the fact that during labour she will not want to eat and, therefore, is not replacing all the vital energy she is using up. As the uterus is a muscle it requires ever-increasing amounts of energy to function efficiently as labour progresses and if it is having to use excess energy. For instance, if the foetus is lying in an awkward position and needs to be rotated before it can progress through the birth canal, it will run out ever sooner.

Should the powers 'decide' to attempt to expel the foetus before the thirty-seventh week of pregnancy, this is classed as a pre-term labour and will need to be managed differently and, in some cases, even stopped. Mum is the best incubator for the foetus and even though the woman may be desperate not to be pregnant anymore, for its overall health and wellbeing, the foetus it is best staying put!!

Another common reason for intervention is going overdue – that is, the pregnancy extending beyond the forty-second week. The main reason for this is that the placenta begins to 'wear out' after this time and, therefore, the risk of lack of oxygen and other vital nutrients to the foetus increases. It is not fully understood whether labour is normally stimulated by the foetus or by the uterus, but in order to stimulate labour it is normal to use a vaginal hormonal pessary and then intravenous synthetic hormones to stimulate the uterus to contract.

An artificially stimulated labour can often be much more painful and violent than a naturally occurring labour and very often both mum and baby are exhausted after the event.

Passages

Basically there are four pelvic shapes. However, it is really only the female gynaecoid pelvis shape that is suited to childbirth. The other shapes have differing inlet, cavity and outlet sizes that are not conducive to the passage of the foetus. Very often it is not until labour that the pelvis is under any sort of 'trial', and not until the passenger has difficulty getting through the passage, that any problems come to light.

This is why it is always a great relief (particularly in a first pregnancy) when the foetal head engages into the inlet of the pelvis. As mentioned before, what goes in will generally come out. So engagement is a very good indicator that the 'passage' is adequate for the passenger. Placental position can affect the 'passage' too in the fact that if it is low-lying and obscuring the internal os then the passenger will not be able to get through without catastrophic consequences so a Caesarean is necessary in this situation.

Passengers

The passenger is obviously the foetus, and the main reason for abnormalities here is the lie of the foetus. For example, if the foetus is lying with its back alongside mum's back it will need to rotate before normal passage and birth can take place. This will require long, strong, effective contractions which are often exhausting. Frequently, the woman will need help with the 'powers' as she expends all her available energy. It is not only the mum that becomes exhausted, though: the foetus can often show signs of not coping with the labour very well – this usually manifests itself in a rise or drop in the heart rate or decelerations after contractions.

Another sign of stress is if the liquor (the water surrounding the foetus in pregnancy) becomes stained with meconium (baby's first stool). This happens because at some point the foetus has suffered a lack of oxygen or a rise in carbon dioxide, for this causes smooth muscle to relax and the foetus to expel the first stool. Another reason is if the foetus is lying in the breech position, that is, with the bottom lying over the internal os instead of the head. The main danger with breech is that whilst the os dilates sufficiently to allow the bottom through, the overall diameter of this part is less than the overall diameter of the skull. This can produce fatal results if the bottom and body have been born but the head cannot get through.

TYPES OF ABNORMAL BIRTH

Tear

This happens when the perineal muscle tears during the final expulsive pushes of the second stage of labour. There are different types of tearing:

First degree: involves the superficial skin of the labia and perineum. Very often does not need stitches.

Second degree: involves the muscle of the perineum and will need suturing to stem the blood flow and aid healing and postnatal repair.

Third degree – involves damage to the anal sphincter and will need suturing (sometimes under general anaesthetic) for effective repair.

Episiotomy

This is a cut made into the perineum by the midwife to widen the passage out for the baby. It is done to avoid sudden tearing, which may result in more damage than an episiotomy, and is made in preparation for the baby's head to come through. An episiotomy is like a second degree tear, in that it will need suturing under sterile conditions.

Vacuum extraction

For vacuum extraction, a small 'skull cap' is placed on the baby's head, a vacuum applied, and then as mum pushes so the doctor pulls and the baby is helped through the final stage of birth.

The most common reason for this is maternal or foetal exhaustion or both, and there is generally great relief all round after the prolonged labour has been bought to an end.

Forceps delivery

This is where the foetus needs a lift out and/or rotation as the head is attempting to pass through the outlet of the pelvis and essentially the woman has become exhausted and is in need of assistance.

The forceps are like large barbeque tools and are placed carefully around the baby's head. Then the doctor pulls while mum pushes. Forceps deliveries including vacuum extraction are usually accompanied by an episiotomy.

Caesarean delivery

In a Caesarean, a surgical incision of approximately six to eight inches (fifteen to twenty centimetres) is made along the bikini line and the foetus is extracted manually. This can be done for a multitude of reasons but the most common is prolonged foetal distress where carbon dioxide levels are rising in the foetal bloodstream and the vital organs of the foetus are seriously under threat. Depending on the severity of the situation, the obstetric team looking after the mother and baby will determine, depending on a number of factors including the severity of the situation, whether a woman requires a spinal or epidural anesthetic.

YOGA WHEN THINGS DON'T GO TO PLAN

During the period that seems 'not to plan', stay with an awareness of your breath moving through your body and feel that the breath can connect you to your baby. You might feel you want to talk to your baby, and share your trust that the best care is being taken of you.

Keep your own authority, listen to your body's response to what is being suggested or asked of you and go with that response. Trust your own inner knowing.

The chapter on postnatal yoga (chapter six, p. 121) gives practices that enable you to recover gradually from any eventuality, so bring those in when you feel ready.

One procedure to avoid at all costs if possible, is being laid flat on your back, with your feet in stirrups, as the after-effects are tremendous pain in the pelvis, especially the pubic bone.

I am amazed this is still done but it happened to one of my students recently, which is why I am mentioning it here. This position causes gravity to push too much force into the pubic bone when it is softening and opening for the baby to come down the birth canal. It also strains the pelvis and all the pelvic muscles as they are very pliable at this stage of labour. They take a long time to recover from this.

It is also totally disenabling to the mother and baby, as they cannot do anything in that position. A squat is much better if at all possible.

If it does happen to you, very careful gentle yoga given in the postnatal section does help recovery but also the pain tends to get better once you stop breastfeeding, because of the hormone change at that stage.

Yoga in its many forms and shapes can be practised at any time in our life in awareness of body, mind and spirit – the word 'mindfulness' is used for this in the Buddha's teaching. Awareness of breath and awareness of body will be enormously helpful to you during labour, whatever path it takes for you, so do remember this.

You may particularly want to have CDs or Ipod tracks of chanting and breath instructions beside you at the time of labour, plus all the things you might normally use in your yoga practice to remind you of the ritual of your practice. It is so important that you have around you who and what you feel at ease with, not worrying about anybody else's ideas of what should or should not be.

Whatever it was like for you can be integrated, healed, absorbed by your yoga practice after the birth, and yet of course you hopefully have a healthy baby which is just one of life's most amazing events and treasures.

If that does not happen for you, know that somewhere in yourself you can accept, understand, go with any eventuality in your life if you have faith in a practice that sustains you. You may find helpful the book A NEW EARTH, by Eckhart Tolle, which focuses on the ego, its role and how we recognize it and see who we really are, helpful especially:

'There are many accounts of people who experienced an emerging new dimension of consciousness as a result of tragic loss at some point in their lives. Some lost all their possessions, others their children or spouse, their social position, reputation or physical abilities.

'In some cases, through disaster or war, they lost all of these simultaneously and found themselves with "nothing". Whatever they had identified with, whatever gave them a sense of self, had been taken away. Then suddenly and inexplicably, the anguish or intense fear they initially felt gave way to a sacred sense of Presence, a deep peace and serenity and complete freedom from fear. It is indeed a peace that doesn't seem to make sense, and the people who experienced it asked themselves: In the face of all this, how can it be that I feel such peace?

'Whenever tragic loss occurs, you either resist or yield. Some people become bitter or deeply resentful; others become compassionate, wise, loving. Yielding means inner acceptance of what is. You are open to life.'

The practice of yoga does, ultimately, bring this about, and so too in my experience does the contact with a new life, especially at the time of birth, even if that new life decides it is not the right time for the journey.

THE FIRST STRUCTURE THAT IS FORMED IN THE CHILD'S BODY (WHILE STILL IN THE WOMB) IS THE SPINE. ALL OTHER LIMBS, THE ARMS, LEGS AND HIPS DERIVE FROM IT. IF THE MOVEMENTS YOU DO IN THE DAY ORIGINATE FROM THE SPINE, THEN THE ACTION IS CORRECT. BUT TO DO THIS AND FEEL THE RESULT OF IT TAKES SOME TIME. BABIES' SPINES ARE EXTREMELY SOFT AND LIGHT AND REMAIN SO FOR A VERY LONG TIME.
THE QUADRUPED ANIMALS ELONGATE THEIR SPINE WITH EACH STEP. WE NEED TO DO THE SAME WHILE WALKING OR STANDING; WITH TWO LEGS THIS IS EVIDENTLY MORE DIFFICULT, BUT, AFTER ALL IT IS ONLY A QUESTION OF STRETCHING OUR KNEES FROM THE HEELS, KEEPING THE HEELS IN CONTACT WITH THE GROUND.
THE ADULT SPINE IS RIGID AND HEAVY AND YOGA, AS INTENDED HERE, CONSISTS IN BREAKING BAD HABITS AND IN RE-EDUCATING THE SPINE SO AS TO BRING IT BACK TO ITS ORIGINAL SUPPLENESS.

VANDA SCARAVELLI, AWAKENING THE SPINE

6. Afterwards: the Postnatal Stage

WE HAVE arrived! To many, congratulations, cards, flowers, good wishes, joy and wonder plus sleepless nights, concern over whether we are doing it right, and an overwhelming number of demands and cares. What now?

BONDING WITH YOUR BABY

The initial few postnatal hours and days, soon to become months, are a crucial time for you, your baby and the baby's father, and any others involved in the care of the baby. There is much talked about bonding at this stage and its importance. If you have tuned into your baby in meditation and breathing as suggested, and bonded with the foetus all through pregnancy, by the

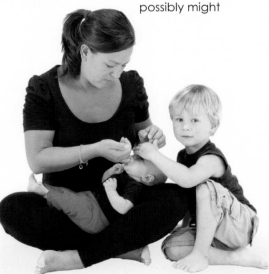

time the baby is born you will feel that bond very strongly. I certainly did! I know my sister, who bonded immediately with her three babies, was concerned that I possibly might

not be so able to bond as I had had a Caesarean and was going to be a single mother, and she was delighted when she saw, after Beth had been taken away for an hour or two to have her heart checked, that I welcomed her back into my arms wholeheartedly.

I can remember just wanting to sit with her in my arms for hours and felt an enormous wrench when she was taken away at all. This may not always be the case at first: I read an article in a newspaper recently by a woman who took several years to feel that deep love for and connection with her child. This can bring an enormous sense of guilt, but is understandable in terms of what we may have been through and the responsibility we now find ourselves with. Also, there may be reasons from our own early life – our mother not bonding with us is the most obvious one, or us not

THE DIVINE ABIDING PARAMETERS – KEY CONCEPTS FOR MEDITATION

APARIGRAHA	Non-possessivenes of people and material things
SANTOSA	Contentment in all circumstances of life. Seeing those circumstances as just what are needed for our soul understanding
KARUNA	Compassion for all, most especially ourselves
MUDITA	Sympathetic joy for the joy and good fortune of others
METTA	Universal love that does not depend on another's attitude to you
UPPEKA	Equanimity in all situations in life

receiving the love we needed, so finding it difficult to give.

Patanjali's sutras in yoga philosophy and the Buddha's teaching can be very helpful in taking us through this time. In particular, the teaching can be helpful if we have looked at and meditated on the concepts in the table above.

If we have been on the lifelong journey to integrate these wonderful principles into our daily awareness, then that experience will take us through many of the difficulties with which this time presents us. One of the remarkable developments in this time is the sense of protection for the child we have given birth to. An analogy that the Buddha made for practitioners on the path is in the phrase, 'As a mother protects with her life her child, her only child'. This quite early becomes apparent, but the intensity and reality of it became clear to me when Panna, one of the students and models in this book, was in a car. Her son was in the passenger seat and she was in the back, not driving, when a car came too near from the side, and she threw herself into the small gap between the baby and the van door. It so much brought home to her the Buddha's words that she could not rest until she had bought a car with three seats in the front.

It is said that a mother could lift a car if her child was underneath it. Where does that incredible strength and determination come from? Such a moment may be the very time that bonding takes place, if it has not yet happened. We become aware of the vast protectiveness that is needed.

SPECIAL DELIVERIES

The possibility that your baby will not be normal, or 'all right', is a great fear for all expectant parents. It can be a torment during pregnancy and heartbreaking after the birth. It can cause mothers and fathers to reject the baby. If we are again to use yoga philosophy, then to feel that this baby may have come for a special reason to special parents, who in some way can manage it, may be the only helpful way to look at what has come about – although it may not seem like it at first, when there is enormous shock and disappointment.

These babies, especially in my experience those with Down's syndrome and cerebral palsy (see p. 26), have enormous love to give and can develop that quality within us. I remember the recent photographs of the UK Conservative Party leader David Cameron with his son Ivan, who had severe epilepsy and cerebral palsy and died in February 2009.

The love and compassion was tangible in those photos. On the other hand, I do know a father who was completely destroyed by the abnormality in his son; the death of that son two years later led him to alcoholism and an accident that has left him paraplegic. Would the practice of yoga here (or, for that matter Buddhism or Christianity) have made a difference to him?

We shall never know: it is incredibly hard caring for a child that is impaired in any way. So much depends on the ability of the parents to surrender to this happening in their lives. These children must have come to teach us, or to allow us to experience something deeper and greater in life. Those four divine abidings of the Buddha, *karuna, mudita, metta* and *uppeka*, in the table opposite, could be of great suppport here. You may like to check the resources on p. 156, too.

EMOTIONAL TRAUMA

Life events such as trauma in childhood (including abuse, the breakdown of their relationship with the baby's father, and worries about money or housing) all can impact on a woman's sense of wellbeing. The tremendous changes associated with childbirth can also unexpectedly bring up strong negative feelings about the loss of an earlier child or a termination or the death of a close family member. Some women find themselves experiencing a grieving process, especially if they were unable to grieve at the time.

This can be very confusing and distressing, at what should be a happy and fulfilling time in a woman's life.

CRYING BABY

Occasionally, despite the parents' best efforts, a baby may still cry and be hard to settle. It is important for women to discuss their difficulties especially if they are getting very tired. Sources of help and support are the Health Visitor or General Practitioner, out-of-hours services or postnatal support groups (see p. 156). Baby massage often helps and sometimes just asking someone to help walking with the baby when they are unsettled is all that is needed.

MIDWIFERY NOTES
ON THE POSTNATAL PERIOD

The postnatal period is defined as the period from which the baby, placenta and membranes have been delivered through to six weeks after. This is when it is generally accepted that the woman's body has returned to 'normal', although in my experience this moment can vary enormously, depending on the woman's birth experience and her support in the immediate postnatal period.

UTERUS AND VAGINAL FLUID-LOSS

Immediately after birth, the uterus shrinks rapidly and the bleeding is stopped by the uterus contracting in on itself and the placental site sealing, while the hormone oxytocin is secreted from the pituitary gland to act upon the uterine muscle. This process, called involution, continues rapidly over the next few days with more and more involution occurring each day until the uterus is back to a pre-pregnant state and not palpable as it is now above the *symphisis pubis*. During this ten-day period the colour of the blood-loss changes from bright red in the first day or two to reddy brown and then to a clearish fluid. If all of the products of conception have not been expelled during the birth process this is the time when infection may start up.

PERINEUM

This is a hugely personal area and women's perception of pain and trauma vary enormously. It is vitally important to be aware of her birth experience, as to whether she sustained a tear, episiotomy or both, and to enquire as to her perception of the healing process and how things are for her now.

Immediately following the birth there will be some pain and discomfort which can be eased by warm baths, bidets, pain relief and gentle exercise. As the days go on this should ease, and as bowel- and bladder-function return to normal so healing is promoted. By six weeks postnatal, most healing should have taken place and sometimes intercourse if she can find a minute!

With some very tactful investigation indeed, it may be possible to find out if there are any minor disorders of the urinary and bowel system. This is incredibly common, although still a difficult area for women to discuss. Again, gentle stretching exercises can be profoundly helpful at this period for what is a distressing problem.

PELVIC FLOOR

There is much discussion as to the benefit of pelvic floor exercises. It is an age-old midwifery norm to advise and encourage women to do the allocated sheet of pelvic floor exercises even though in yoga terms these tend to be quite forced and unnatural. More recently, particularly, I have had to acknowledge that my experience is that a more natural, less forced, more of a 'stretching' approach is more successful and less rigid and painful.

BREASTS

After the birth the levels of progesterone and oestrogen drop and levels of the hormone prolactin increase, causing the production of milk. The hormone oxytocin controls the ejection of the milk. Colostrum is the name given to the milk produced in the first twenty-four to forty-eight hours. This is very high in protein and immunoglobulins, and so protects the newborn from infection in the early days. Also this will sustain the baby initially as it

has high levels of residual fat laid down in the latter weeks of pregnancy to ensure it survives the crucial period around the time of birth. On day three or four, the baby's needs change, and he or she requires a more sustaining feed, so the milk becomes much higher in fat; women will describe a feeling of incredible fullness. It will be obvious that the milk has 'come in'.

Although a great many of the available publications make breastfeeding look the most natural thing in the world, in my experience many women do not find it at all easy and need to know that it takes time, lots of patience and most of all a relaxed approach – which can be really challenging if the baby is impatient and not particularly relaxed!

Good posture while breastfeeding is all-important, too, right from the outset, to avoid upper back ache, and undue strain on the lower back. So if it takes a few extra minutes to get really comfortable, this is really worthwhile. The mother could be feeding for anything up to an hour at a time initially, so any investment in time and positioning is a very good idea.

URDHVA DANDASANA (SEE P. 135) IS A GOOD POSTURE IN WHICH TO RESTORE ENERGIES, REST TIRED LEGS AND TAKE A BREATHER.
USE A CHAIR TO PUT THE LEGS ON IF THIS IS MORE COMFORTABLE

THE CIRCULATORY SYSTEM

Following the birth, the body has to reabsorb a quantity of fluid. This results in the woman passing large and frequent amounts of urine during the first few days after the birth. This fluid may also accumulate in the ankles and calves resulting in swelling in these areas.

Gentle exercise and no standing for prolonged periods of time is the normal advice, along with 'marching on the spot' if the mother is stationary for any length of time – for instance, when attending to the baby. After not standing for long periods, the posture on the previous page will help; alternatively, do the modified standing postures on pp. 147–8).

Yoga
Move in and out of standing poses quite quickly to help circulation in legs, and then, lie with legs up the wall or on a chair. (Do not do these until six months after the birth if you have had tearing or an episiotomy.)

THE MUSCULOSKELETAL SYSTEM

As mentioned, as soon as the baby, placenta and membranes are delivered the levels of progesterone and oestrogen drop off. Gradually, joints and ligaments will return to a pre-pregnant state but this can take up to three months in some women and during this time the muscles and ligaments are susceptible to pain and injury, so you need to be aware of how they move and careful of how they lift (their baby for example)

Yoga
Lie on your back with your legs up the wall or on a chair or stool.

THE DIGESTIVE SYSTEM

Initially, and much to her delight, a mother can lose anything up to 5kg in weight immediately after the birth, and see her toes again!!! In my experience it takes nine months to build a baby and nine months to get rid of the excess weight. There is a huge amount of pressure on women to get back to their pre-pregnant state quickly, very often at the expense of themselves and their breastfeeding. While feeding, it is essential the mother eats enough calories to provide strong milk for the baby, so she needs to maintain a really adequate intake to do this and do her very best to forget about wanting to be stick-thin within a few weeks.

One common postnatal complaint can be the presence of haemorrhoids. These can persist often for months after the birth and be really troublesome.

Yoga
Twists as given in this chapter (below, p. 142).

THE RESPIRATORY SYSTEM

The respiratory system returns to normal very soon after the birth, usually accompanied by much relief on the woman's part that she can breathe well again.

BREASTFEEDING

Notes contributed by Inner Yoga teacher Joy Hosie

'Breastfeeding is an art rather than a science. You can read as many books and listen to as many midwives or experienced mothers as you like, but the reality is that every woman's breasts and baby are unique to them. There is a symbiotic relationship between the mother, baby and milk production which can only be learned and understood on an individual level – which in turn requires patience and awareness.

'Since neither the breasts nor the baby's digestive system are transparent, the only thing you can do is trust your instincts in relation to breastfeeding and try not to get too wound up about it. In the early days this can sometimes be easier said than done. When your baby is screaming with hunger (sometimes it is just a desire to communicate and not quite as alarming as it can sound at first) and you yourself are tired, it is all the more important to prepare yourself (as one would always) in a yogic approach and to try to centre yourself. The desire to nourish your new baby is usually overwhelming, but the ability to breastfeed doesn't come easily to every woman. In fact most women, if they are honest, will find some difficulty particularly with their first baby. It can also depend on what type of birth experience you yourself have had, how much blood you have lost and generally how you are in yourself post-birth.

'In addition, there is a significant shift in hormones after the birth which can be difficult to adjust to and the mother can often feel anxious, tearful or lacking in confidence if the breastfeeding is not going as well as anticipated.

'In the early days, the positioning in order to breastfeed is vital. At its best the pouring forth of milk and love from the heart centre to your new offspring is not that easy to achieve when you have a tiny wriggling screaming being who may or may not know how to suckle effectively – and you are tired or overwhelmed by it all. This can be particularly challenging if you have sore or cracked nipples, which in the early days is more often the case than not.

'Take heart, though, as it is a bit like driving. A lot of preparation is required in the learning stages, and it all seems so difficult but there is a time when it all just clicks into place and you are able to do it naturally and almost without thinking too much about it. Breastfeeding is similar. Although the umbilical cord is cut after the birth, there is still very much a spiritual cord between the mother and baby and it feels as if mother and baby are still connected.

'This feeling can be so strong that it feels almost a physical one. If your baby is crying and hungry, it is like having a pain in your own body. You just want it to be taken away and for the pain to stop. It is really important at this stage to broaden your awareness in terms of that sense of pain and to centre yourself, moving with awareness, to get yourself into the correct position. Tightening the body in response or looking for a quick fix will not help.

'Prepare yourself and your body, however loudly your wee one is screaming. Communicate with your baby and tell her or him that you understand that she or he is hungry and that you will feed him or her. Responding to the baby's needs by communicating verbally all assists in the development of the mother–baby bond, and eventually the baby will respond by being soothed by the mother's voice and her energy.

'Sit comfortably, preferably in a low position, to allow the opening and spreading of the sacrum. Try to avoid sitting on bucket-shaped seats or sofas. Make sure you have appropriate support at your back so that the pelvis is tipped forward slightly, allowing spreading and opening from the base.

'Use the breath to take your awareness to the base and try to open and spread there. Breathe into the back of the body and the lumbar area. Make sure you have cushions or pillows to support the baby on so that the baby is at the correct height for access to your breasts.

'It is worth taking time to tune in with your own body's needs and to make yourself comfortable, as ultimately this will be what is necessary for the baby too. Most women adopt hunched up postures when breastfeeding, resulting in aching backs, shoulders and necks. Poor posture can also result in lactation problems in the early days of breastfeeding when you are trying to ensure that the baby is properly latched on and suckling well.

'Position the baby on cushions on your lap and bend forward as if to do a seated *Paschimottanasana*, keeping the knees soft and open to avoid putting too much strain on any injuries which are healing. Try to tune into your own breath as much as possible.

'With your hands underneath the cushions, scoop the baby up on an inbreath and exhale to spread into the base to raise yourself back up to a seated posture. Bend forward once again from the base as if in modified *Paschimottanasana* in order to latch your baby on.

'This forward-bending movement is helpful in order to achieve a good latch. It is particularly important in large-breasted women who cannot see what the baby's bottom lip is doing. The lip needs to be soft and as much of the whole nipple and areola as possible in the baby's mouth, with the tip of the nipple pointing up to the roof of the baby's mouth. It is much easier to do this when you are bending forward but somewhat counterproductive if you are stiff in the base and hunched over in the back and shoulders.

'If the baby is not latched on properly and the breast not adequately drained of milk, mastitis can occur, requiring treatment with antibiotics and often hospitalization. Even later on, once you become an accomplished expert in breastfeeding and are more comfortable in the baby latching on properly, it is still important to avoid shoulder, neck and back strain.

'Once you know the baby is latched on properly then you can scoop the baby up again and move to a more upright position where you can relax and allow the shoulders to drop and the back of the body to relax.

'In the early days of breastfeeding, it can sometimes be painful to feed, particularly if you have cracked or sore nipples. The tendency can then be to hunch the shoulders and recoil from the pain. It is good at this stage (after checking that the baby is latched on properly) to take one's awareness to the breath and breathe through any discomfort, encouraging the back to relax and the shoulders to drop.

'Awareness should also be taken to the position of the hands. If you are supporting your baby underneath, then make sure that you have a good spread of the fingers and stretch of the hand from the thumb to the little finger, as this will encourage the shoulderblade to drop and the surrounding muscles to relax and drop taking any strain off the back and neck. In a very young baby you may be supporting their neck and head with your thumb and forefinger.

'Again, try to spread them and the other fingers as much as possible in order to encourage the drop of the shoulderblade and the relaxation of the back muscles.

'Once time and care has been taken to open and spread the body from the base, to latch the baby on and to relax the shoulders, you will find that the head will dip naturally and without strain if focus is maintained on the breath and the *jalandhara bandha* is engaged.

'As well as becoming meditative, you can also keep an eye on your baby from this position without creating strain in the neck and shoulders. '

> YOUR CHILDREN ARE NOT YOUR CHILDREN. THEY ARE THE SONS AND DAUGHTERS OF LIFE'S LONGING FOR ITSELF. THEY CAME THROUGH YOU BUT NOT FROM YOU AND THOUGH THEY ARE WITH YOU YET THEY BELONG NOT TO YOU.
>
> KAHLIL GIBRAN

SUPPORT GROUPS

Your GP surgery or public health nursing team will have information on local supports services or groups to help establish breastfeeding and to meet other breastfeeding mums to share experiences. There are some other addresses on p. 156, too.

RELINQUISHING BREASTFEEDING

For many women, breastfeeding is a rewarding and fulfilling experience However, for some, and for a wide variety of reasons, that is not the case and breastfeeding does not happen. In my experience it is important for these women to remember that there are many ways to show their love and care for their baby and to share intimate moments without breastfeeding.

Trying to make sensible decisions and not being left with a residue of guilt is difficult but very important. Mothers who cannot breastfeed their first child may go on to find they can feed subsequent babies. As with many issues, in the complex skill of parenting some things will go smoothly, while others will not be possible at that time.

POSTNATAL DEPRESSION

Postnatal 'blues' are experienced by between half and three-quarters of women who have given birth, usually on day three or four after the birth. They often describe it in terms of feeling tearful, depressed and withdrawn. This is usually only a temporary situation that lifts after a day or so. It is thought to occur as progesterone and oestrogen drop off, prolactin kicks in and the breasts fill with milk.

Another reason for postnatal 'blues' and distress can be birth events themselves. Very often not living up to the woman's hopes and expectations, she can feel she has let herself down and can easily feel a failure if she hasn't been able to achieve what she set out to achieve. In my experience in the antenatal period it is so important not to get hooked on outcomes and to remain open-minded.

Mild to moderate postnatal depression has a later onset than baby 'blues' and is more chronic, manifesting itself in feelings of inability to cope, feelings of being overwhelmed by the new responsibility

and sleep disturbances. In the UK, around the tenth day the midwife hands on care to the Health Visiting Team (sometimes called Public Health Nurses). The Public Health Nurse will make contact and arrange to meet the family and the new baby to support and discuss any issues or concerns including any worries about physical or mental wellbeing. Public health nurses are generally based at GP surgeries. Around six to eight week after delivery a health check is offered for both the woman and the baby.

This will include screening for postnatal depression and is a good opportunity for women to discuss with the HV or GP how they are feeling.

One in ten women get mild to moderate postnatal depression. It is most commonly resolved with counselling and expert discussion.

Severe depressive illness can manifest some two to three weeks after the birth, and there will be greater sleep disturbance, impaired concentration and lack of ability to cope with everyday life. This can be accompanied by weight loss, feelings of guilt and incompetence and delusional thoughts. This needs expert

help with counselling, antidepressants and careful follow-up. The key to early intervention, which will alleviate the longterm impact on the woman and her family, is for her to tell someone how she is feeling, but this may seem almost impossible when she is depressed. Those around the mother and baby are often those who pick up the changes and should have the information and feel able to discuss their concerns with the woman and the professionals involved.

Puerperal psychosis is the most serious form of postnatal depression and generally leads to psychiatric admission to a mother and baby unit as she could be a danger to herself and to her baby. This manifests itself early in the postnatal period with severe mood changes, irrational behaviour, disturbed agitated actions, hallucinations and she obviously begins to lose touch with reality. There may be no history of mental illness and it can be terrifying for her partner especially as the onset is early and generally so sudden. With the right treatment this is totally curable although she would need to be referred for medical help in her next pregnancy as it could easily occur again.

Yoga for postnatal depression (except for puerperal psychosis)

Yoga in all its aspects would be very supportive in postnatal depression, particularly where you take the spine back into an arch such as *Setu Bandha Sarvangasana* (Bridge pose), *Supta virasana* (going back in Hero); also *Salamba sarvangasana* (Shoulderstand) and *Uttanasana* (Standing Forward Bend).

It can be an enormous challenge to get yourself to do any yoga at all – so a little, even two minutes to start with would be helpful. Sometimes meditation does not feel helpful as too much can come up in thoughts. Either leave it for the moment or move in it – backwards, forwards and twisting the spine on its axis.

In the photos, see how Tamsin is lifting her arms out to the side and twisting the spine. She then repeats the twist with one arm on her knee and one behind to take the spine around further. This movement of the spine on its axis lifts the energy and spirits.

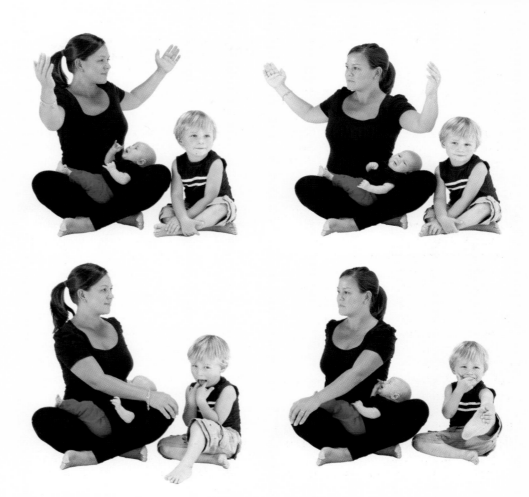

POSTNATAL YOGA

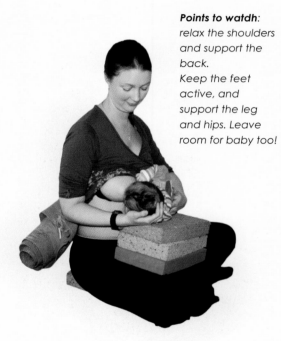

Points to watdh:
relax the shoulders and support the back.
Keep the feet active, and support the leg and hips. Leave room for baby too!

Although from a medical perspective Sally gives the postnatal period as six weeks, as far as yoga is concerned the time given is two years – a big difference! This is more the Indian way, giving time for the shift of hormones, the change in the body and the psyche of the mother. It is an enormous adjustment, as was the shift of the body to the pregnant state.

So although you might get back to your normal yoga practice much quicker than that, remember that your body needs gentle care and consideration.

These first few postures on the shoulders and upper back can be done soon after the birth as it is that part of the body that feels under strain, from heavy breasts, possibly breastfeeding and holding your baby, or even two babies!

SITTING FOR BREASTFEEDING AND MEDITATION

I found breastfeeding, once I had got used to it and my nipples had recovered, a wonderful chance to sit, be quiet, contemplate and meditate. It is a very calm meditative time that connects you to your baby, to enhance that lifelong link.

My colleague, Joy Hosie, has already contrbuted some notes on breastfeeding to this book (pp 127–9), but here is my personal experience. If you are comfortable, sit cross-legged. If you have had any tearing or episiotomy or do not easily sit cross-legged, or in illness or discomfort, either sit in *Virasana*, Hero pose, or on a low chair, for a three- to six-month period, or sit on a settee, futon or the floor with some support for your back. In the photo on the left, Paula is sitting with her back against the wall and a rolled blanket supporting her lower back, which has the effect of allowing the upper back to lift up and over the support. Put two or three cushions or pillows on your lap so that the baby is at the right height for you, then breastfeeding will be relaxed for both of you.

Gradually settle into a quiet meditative space, aware of your breathing, aware of your contented baby and appreciate this very precious time, a time you will

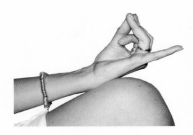

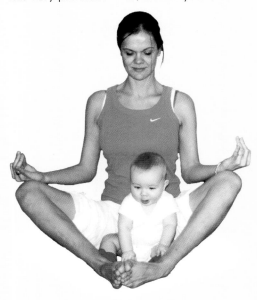

remember all through your baby's life. I found the first feed of the morning was the best time of the day, as you were fresher and the baby settled. I also used to breastfeed at the end of a yoga class while I was talking people through relaxation. Perhaps it had an effect on my baby and me?

It is helpful while you are sitting here, or while you are able to have a few minutes of meditation, to use the *Hridaya mudra* shown in the small picture. 'Hridaya' means heart, and the mudra connects us back to our heart space or centre and brings calm and understanding to the mind and body.

Especially helpful in all situations in life but particularly if we feel upset or cross with our children or find them too much at any given time, it gives us a bigger

picture of the whole of life.

In that meditative space tune in to your own inner knowing, so that you will know what is best for this child from your own inner connection. From the time they were in your womb and now in their total dependency on you, feel the privilege and honour of that.

There will be many times when you want to run away from this vitally important job given to you, many times when you will want to tear your hair out, feel furious with your child, but if you can be in acceptance of all those understandable feelings that well up now it will stand you in good stead as you go through their life.

As Beth reaches the stage of late teenage, I find myself regretting the time I did not spend with my baby and child. This is very hard to deal with, and common to many parents, I think. One reason that we want to get away is that it all feels too much to deal with and we do not know if we are doing all right with it, or doing it 'right'. No one can tell us this, we need have faith in ourselves and the role we have been given. This is where grandparents are wonderful; they have been through the whole process. They can and will deal with it all in its vastness and make such a special link to your child, that your child usually responds to immediately. Perhaps one thing we can look forward to when at last we become a grandparent is to be able to heal any regret we may feel around our relationship to our own children. I look forward to that.

After this breastfeeding meditation, put your baby down to sleep or relax contentedly and rather than being tempted to rush around 'doing things, catching up' do the next few postures, as you will really feel the benefit of them in your day; they will relax you yet wake you up, to a much greater efficiency and enjoyment of your day. They only need take five to ten minutes – you can give yourself that!

There is a tendency in our culture, especially when we are parents, to feel

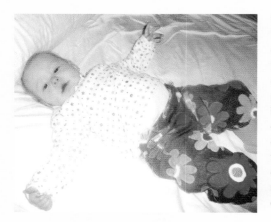

WATCH YOUR BABY. SEE HOW RELAXED HE OR SHE IS WHEN RESTING OR SLEEPING OR HAPPY

that any time spent on ourselves is selfish. We think that we should be spending it on others, work, housework etc. However, time spent on and with ourselves enhances our own self and our life, and makes such a difference to our day that it makes a difference to all with whom we come into contact. We will have more energy, more awareness of others and their needs, more understanding and compassion for others and, especially, more imaginative understanding of our children.

PRECAUTIONS IN POSTNATAL YOGA

1. Do not do anything that pulls or strains the pelvic floor and abdominal area.
2. Do not overdo or push yourself but do give yourself some time to be with yourself.

1. Urdhva Dandasana
REVERSE STAFF POSE WITH LEGS UP THE WALL

Points to watch: *rest the shoulderblades down and spread the shoulders. Rest the abdominal muscles back and in the version on the right spread the feet onto the wall*

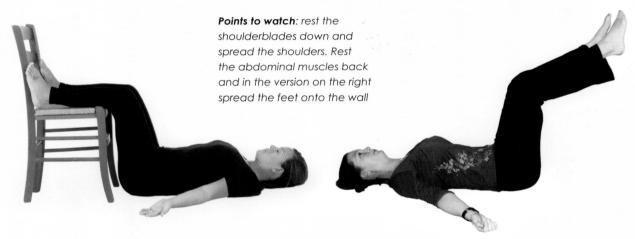

Find a spare piece of wall, as Panna has in the righthand photo, or if this pose is too much for your hamstrings or back, copy Tamsin in using a chair to put your legs on (lefthand picture). Rest your arms overhead where comfortable or to the side if that pulls any where.

Relax there breathing into your back ribs, which is much easier in this position. Feel your shoulderblades and upper spine drop back gradually onto the ground, and your throat and neck relax. This time is very demanding on your body, as was pregnancy, and you need to take care of yourself, both for yourself and for all your family. When it feels enough roll over to one side to come up from your side to sitting, or go on to *Salamba sarvangasana*, Shoulderstand, overleaf.

2. SALAMBA SARVANGASANA
SUPPORTED SHOULDERSTAND USING THE WALL

Points to watch: *spread the shoulders down and the feet onto the wall*

Points to watch: *lift only as far as you can go without a tightening in the back. The thighs lengthen up out of the hips. Spread the heels into the wall with the shins working, so that the legs lift you.*

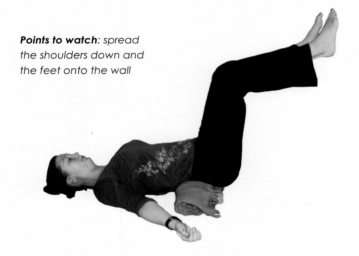

You may feel, after you have been with your legs up and feet on the wall for a few minutes, that you want to bend your knees, putting your feet on the wall, to go towards a supported Shoulderstand. I wanted to do this very soon after my Caesarean (making sure I did not extend over the scar) as it was so re-energizing. If you have had any stitching, do not let it pull at all for three months.

Use your feet and legs to lift your back off the ground. You may then want to put a block or two and a rolled blanket, as shown, under your back and rest there in *Viparita karani* (Reversing attitude), or lengthen up through one leg by taking the opposite foot firm into the wall. Then you will find that both legs will work for you more and your knees can move up towards the ceiling, giving gradually more lift on your back. When you are ready to come down, bend your knees and roll onto one side, resting there for a minute. Come up from your side to sitting.

This sequence restores your energy, revitalizes your legs, prevents and relieves varicose veins. It brings all things in life into perspective, and calms the mind and emotions.

3. GOMUKASANA
COW FACE POSE

Points to watch: *the elbow rests in the palm, and the shoulders are rested down*

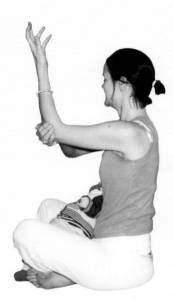

Points to watch: *see how Paula's chest is spreading*

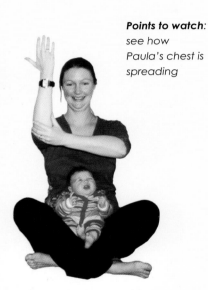

Points to watch: *see how Paula's upper arm is rolled in and up to spread the shoulders. Lower the other elbow, easing the back down.*

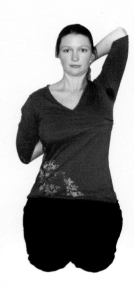

Sitting in *Virasana* (Hero pose), or simply cross-legged, on a block or cushion or two, lengthen your arms forward to shoulder height, relaxing your shoulderblades down your back, let your arms move up over your head, ease up out of one hip and then the other, so that you are moving from the lower ribs where the muscles of the arms insert onto the bone.

Take hold of one elbow as shown and bring your hand onto the base of the neck, relax your upper arm into your shoulder joint, as you lift your elbow up above your shoulder. Repeat on the other side.

Do the same again, and when you have the upper arm in place bring the lower arm around across the back ribs, resting there a moment to feel the breath in the back of the body, then gently ease the arm up the upper back, spreading your upper back and neck vertebrae into your hand and wrist. Do not strain to touch the hands (see how Tamsin has them in the middle picture). Touching does not matter, it's the release and spread given in the shoulders and upper back that feels so good at this stage when you are constantly holding the baby and feeding.

Then undo the arms and repeat on the other side.

Points to watch: *spread your hand into the base of neck and the neck back into the arm. Ease the elbow up and back with your other hand*

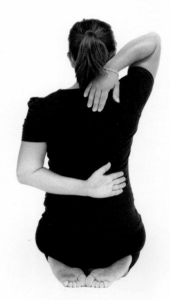

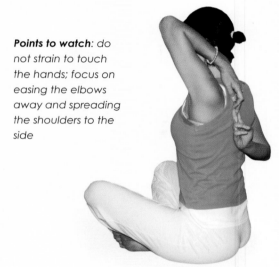

Points to watch: *do not strain to touch the hands; focus on easing the elbows away and spreading the shoulders to the side*

4. PARSVA NAMASTE
PRAYER POSE BEHIND YOUR BACK

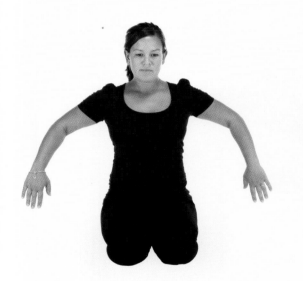 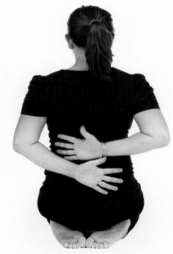 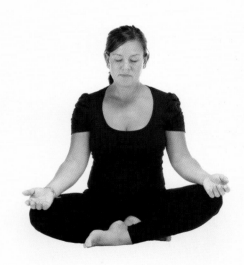

Ease your elbows out to the side. This reminds me of cormorants as they hang their wings out to dry. Bring your elbows back, loosely clasp your hands behind you, and

ease back through one shoulder then the other. You can then rest your lower arms on your back ribs, enjoying the spread across your chest and release in your shoulders.

If and when you feel ready, ease your fingertips together. Turn them up towards your head to bring them into a prayer position, spreading them into your upper back.

Open out through your elbows to spread your breastbone without pushing your chest forward as this will strain your back. Gently undo your hands. Go on to the next pose.

5. PINDASANA
CHILD OR EMBRYO POSE

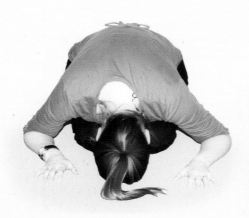 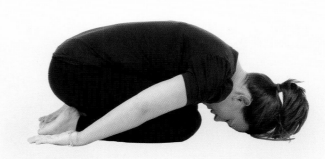

Take your spine forward over your legs, your crown spreading down towards the ground, your arms resting down beside your head (left picture). Feel the spread of your ribs onto your legs as you breathe from your diaphragm, opening out across the collarbone as the breath comes up to your top chest, or relax your arms back down by your side, making sure that the neck is not crushed at all. Ease down through your legs back through your base to come up to sitting, ease forward onto all fours to stretch your legs back behind you one at a time. Then stretch your legs forward into *Dandasana* (Staff pose), spreading your fingertips to lengthen your spine up.

This sequence relieves any strain in your spine and shoulders, opens your heart area, lifts your energy, and relaxes a busy, overdone mind. If you have had a straightforward labour with no intervention, then you can go straight onto the next postures.

6. RESTORATION OF THE PELVIC FLOOR,
USING MULA BANDHA MUDRA

Remember that the principle while you were pregnant was to broaden down and out towards the base of your spine, to help and encourage the direction the baby was going to take. Now, to restore the balance in your pelvis, you are moving your energy in and up. This is a subtle movement of the inner body and inner energy (see 'Pelvic Floor', p. 125), not the tightening, forceful contraction of many traditional pelvic-floor exercises (I haven't met a woman yet who felt like doing those exercises after giving birth). So trust that awareness or inner knowing; it will be very strong in you at this time.

The pelvic floor will restore itself through breastfeeding, and also through breathing from the thoracic and pelvic-floor diaphragms (see pp. 12–13)

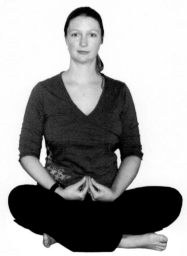

which work together; when one moves the other must follow. Engaging this inner awareness of the energy doming up in the base area, and arching out in the solar plexus area, helps to restore the pelvic floor to its natural state. This

movement in the base is called *Mula bandha* (see p. 14).

Sit in any comfortable posture so that your hands can rest on your lap. Bring the index finger to touch the pad of the thumb, and bring the other fingers in line with the index finger, all touching one another. Make each fingernail touch the fingernail of the opposite hand and ease the fingers upwards, to form Hasta mudra, as illustrated here. It is a version of *Brahman mudra*, but I have termed it *Mula bandha mudra*. The mudras work subtly, the nerve endings from the hands and feet connecting with the whole body. Here there is a subtle feeling in the breath body – the doming in and up of the *Mula bandha* across the pelvic floor. The awareness in the thoracic diaphragm is the *Uddiyhana*

bandha, meaning 'to fly up'.

All the following postures have that awareness of energy moving in and up through the spine, and being contained there. This is my understanding of the basic principle in Vanda Scaravelli's teaching of asanas in AWAKENING THE SPINE. They will specifically work on the pelvic floor when practised in this way, moving from the base of the spine upwards – but note that initially you may not feel the effect of this bandha if you haven't done much yoga before as it is subtle, but your awareness will increase, in both the postures and breathing, with practice.

The twists on the following pages can particularly have this movement of coming in and up through the spine. You can now gradually introduce all postures, applying this same principle.

7. MARICHYASANA III
SAGE MARICHI'S POSES

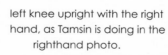

From *Dandasana*, Staff pose (picture below), bend up your left knee, and take your left fingertips onto ground behind you.

Spread the left foot firmly into the ground and feel the spine lengthen up and spiral to the left. As you spiral the spine, keep the

strong flat tendon that runs from the inner heel to the ball of the foot and then out over the backs of the toes, connects to the pelvic floor and thoracic diaphragm. When the arch of the foot is working then these diaphragms are working.)

left knee upright with the right hand, as Tamsin is doing in the righthand photo.

Now loop the elbow around the knee as Saskia is doing (above) to increase the twist of the spine. Go on extending into both heels, as this brings the pelvic floor in and up in a firm yet gentle way.

The aponeurosis plantar, the

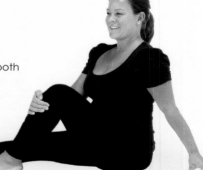

8. MARICHYASANA I
SAGE MARICHI'S POSES

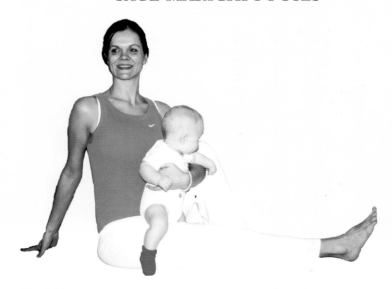

In this twist, bend up the left knee.

Take the right hand behind and the left arm against the left leg so that the left foot, going firmly down, lifts the spine and twists it to the right.

In the picture, Saskia is standing down on her left foot to lengthen up her spine, and so spiral it around to her right. The way she is holding Sam is actually helping this movement and lift her up through the breastbone. There is room for baby Sam to sit, and so to relax the leg down.

Repeat, turning to the other side.

You can do many of these poses with your baby around you.

9. PASCHIMOTTANASANA
SITTING FORWARD BEND

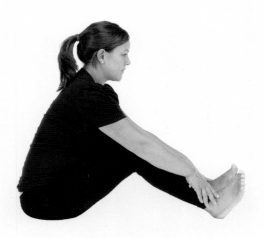

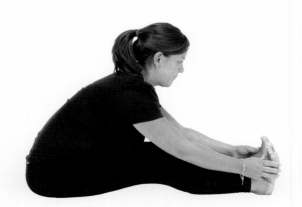

After *Marichyasana*, bring both heels onto the ground (left photo) and then, keeping the spine extending up, extend the heels away along the ground. Bring the arms forward but keep the shoulders relaxed back and down. Now walk the thighs back into the hips, first one side and then the other (righthand picture), lengthening the spine forward and up.

If it makes your back ache generally all over, that's because you are waking up the back, but do not hold the posture too long, and relax afterwards, lying down on your back with your legs elevated as shown, in the pose on the front cover known as *Supta vajrasana*, named 'the little boat' by Vanda Scaravelli.

If it helps the sacrum and therefore the spine to cross your feet at your ankles, with your legs up across your pelvis. Keep your feet working and your heels connected back into your shins and ankles, so that you feel the relief and spread to the sacrum.

Roll to your side when you are ready to come up to sitting and go on to the next pose, *Baddha konasana*.

10. BADDHA KONASANA
COBBLER POSE

Points to watch:
fingers in Hridaya
mudra *(heart mudra)*

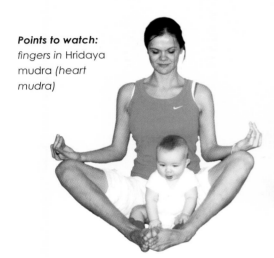

Points to watch:
*a cross-legged
posture is better after
Caesarean section;
sit in Virasana (Hero
pose) if other poses
pull across the scar
at all*

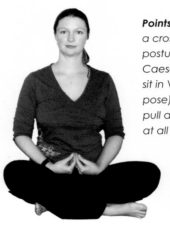

Points to watch:
*note the heels
spreading into
one another*

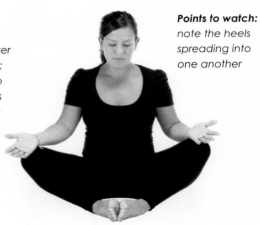

Baddha konasana is demonstrated here first by Saskia, with baby Sam sitting in the same position tucked cosily in by his mum's hips and thighs. Beside them, Paula sits cross-legged, as *baddha konasana* can feel too much for the hips after a Caesarean section. She sits in *mula bandha mudra* (p. 141) to bring the pelvic floor back to its pre-pregnant state.

From Staff pose, bend your knees to bring the soles of your feet together so that your hips open out and therefore your spine can lengthen up out of your hips.

Opening the palms, as in the picture of Tamsin, above right, spreads the thoracic diaphragm to that breathing comes from the the pelvic floor and the thoracic diaphragm. This will help restore the pelvic floor too.

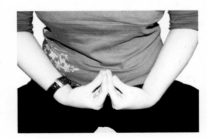

11. Maha Mudra
THE GREAT MUDRA

This posture is in a similar position to *Janu sirsasana* but it is a mudra so you do not go forward.

From *Baddha konasana*, lengthen out the left leg, extend the spine up and around over the straight leg. Place both hands on your leg or either side. From the heels, gather your legs back into your hips and pelvic floor, so that you feel the doming up of the Mula Bandha at the base. Feel this lift the spine up out of the hips so that the ribs open out and fly up into the *Uddiyhana bandha*. This will spread the breastbone, shoulders and upper back, letting the throat relax back into the neck into the *Jalandhara bandha*.

The head then comes down so the neck lengthens and shoulders

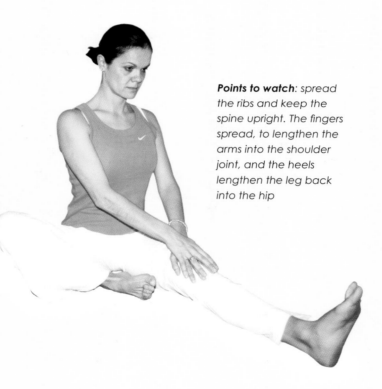

Points to watch: spread the ribs and keep the spine upright. The fingers spread, to lengthen the arms into the shoulder joint, and the heels lengthen the leg back into the hip

broaden again. This could all happen, if you are at ease doing so, on an inhalation. Then gently exhale, maintaining the length of the spine. Take an easy breath in and out before repeating. Then lengthen the leg out and bend the other leg, to repeat on the other side.

Lie down afterwards to relax and rest.

In terms of yoga practice this is more advanced, so if it feels at all a strain, leave it and come back to it later.

It is a powerful posture that energizes and awakens the whole body, especially the spine, employing all the bandhas to contain the energy within the spine.

12. Parsvottanasana to Utthita Parsvakonasana
EXTENDED SIDE STRETCH AND STRETCHED FLANK POSE

'Extended side stretch' is the literal translation of *Parsvottanasana*; I like to call it Egret pose (see p. 56). Egrets are more common in England now, but the egret I saw around the Taj Mahal gave exactly that sense of the lift up into the hips from the legs and feet that is needed in this pose. With knee bent, it becomes *Utthita parsvakonasana* (as shown in the lefthand photo).

Place a chair in front of you, spreading your hands down onto the chair so that your spine comes forward and down. Then step one foot back, spread firmly down through your feet, opening out through your toes and back into your heels to lengthen your spine forward out of your hips.

Points to watch: *lengthen up from the feet to the thighbone to take the spine forward*

Then, bending your front knee, turn your back foot so you lift up into that hip to spiral your spine up and around. Your chest and arm following the movement of your spine. To change to the other side, put the lifted hand back on the chair step the back foot forward and take the front foot back.

This pose will strengthen your legs and spine, and restore the pelvic floor and the digestive system.

Points to watch: *do not lift the arm if the shoulder strains, but keep the hand relaxed on the hip*

13. Parivrtta and Utthita Trikonasana
REVERSE AND STRETCHED TRIANGLE POSES, USING THE WALL

The following standing postures probably need to come later in the postnatal period, especially if there were any complications in childbirth. Until three to six months are up, the sitting and inverted postures will be more restful.

Stand facing the wall, stepping your right foot forward, and bring both hands up onto the wall above your shoulder height, as shown in the first picture.

Spread down into your right foot, and then extend up from your feet to bring your right thighbone into your hip joint. This will move your spine forward, out of your hips, and spiral it around towards your right leg and bring your right shoulder back so that your right hand comes down onto your right hip. This is *Parivrtta trikonasana* (middle picture).

To come out, spread back into your back heel and step that foot forward. Repeat with the other foot and hand.

Now, come back to the pose of the first picture with both hands on the wall and right foot forward.

Spread into the the left heel and up through the thighbone into the left hip, bringing the left hand back onto the left hip. Let the whole spine spiral up and around

on its axis to the left. This is *Utthita trikonasana* (righthand picture). Come back to the original position and bring the left foot forward to change to the other side.

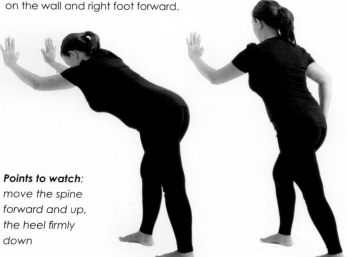

Points to watch: *move the spine forward and up, the heel firmly down*

Points to watch: *spread the heel down to move the thighbone up and back into hip joint, to bring in the* mula bandha *as the pelvic floor domes up*

14. Setu Bandha Sarvangasana
BRIDGE POSE WITH BABY

Points to watch: *feel the spine moving towards the head, the pelvis relaxed and the heels firmly down*

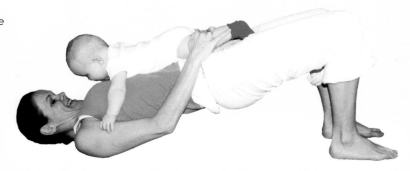

There are many poses where your baby can be around and have fun with you in a pose.

In *Setu bandha sarvangasana* (Bridge pose), if you wish, relax your baby on your tummy as shown, and then, spreading your feet into the ground, lengthen your knees away and down so that your spine moves towards your head and then your pelvis will lift, but do not push your pelvis up as this will tighten your back. Feel the very base of the spine moving towards your head to tone the pelvic floor, broadening out across the pelvis as you do so.

When my daughter was crawling she would have fun crawling backwards and forwards underneath me, and then use my pelvis to get herself up to standing – it was a great game for her. Here baby Sam is enjoying being turned upside down as all babies I have met do.

DAD AND BABY YOGA

Let's not forget what Dad can do – especially if the baby, as Bella is here, has a little snooze at a convenient angle!

Here's what Will wrote about his first experience as a father.

'As a new father I am full of joy watching the development of a new life in all her cheeky and cute ways! As fellow parents will know, babies need much care, attention and patience at all hours, which has placed quite a demand on my energy and made me really value my personal time. Yoga helps me balance these new demands in a number of ways.

'First, and on a very practical level, when feeding Bella I make sure that my lower back is well supported, my torso and hips symmetrical and shoulders open, in order that my upper back doesn't round.

'With so much time spent feeding I find it particularly important to get this position comfortable. Feeding time is also a good opportunity to relax, breathe and meditate. I'm sure Bella benefits energetically from the sense of calm that comes from this.

'In addition, a big help for me is the awareness that yoga and meditation have taught me over the years: lessons in impermanence when crying is prolonged; lessons in 'not taking it personally'; lessons in tolerance, and learning to be with what is and knowing that it will change again.

'My journey into parenting is only just beginning!'

We can learn so much from our children about the body, especially at this age before they sit in chairs, which ruins our posture. We also learn so much about life from our children. They are our greatest teachers: they require our full attention and infinite patience. These are two qualities which perhaps our 'modern, civilized life' has deprived us of, so our children are a good practice ground to regain these qualities which are a strong and important part of the practice of yoga in all its forms and are qualities that both the Christ and the Buddha gave attention to in their teaching.

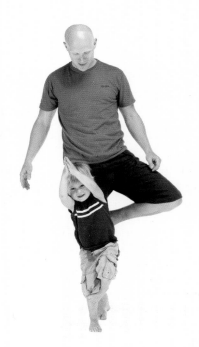

CHRIS IN VRKSASANA, TREE POSE, WITH SAMUEL

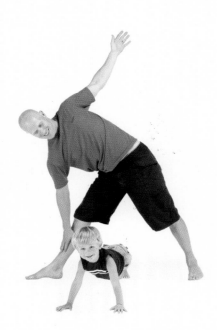

TRIANGLE, WITH SAMUEL IN ADHO MUKA SVANASANA,
FACE-UP DOG POSE

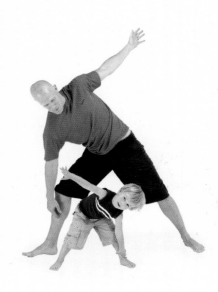

TRIKONASANA, TRIANGLE POSE

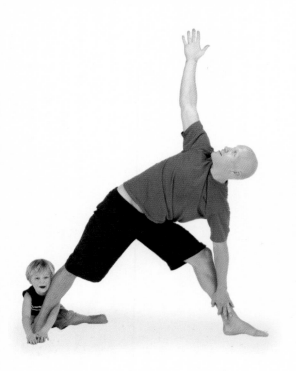

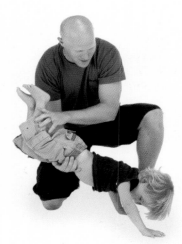

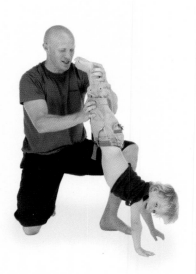

HELPING IN UTTHITA PARSVAKONASANA,
STRETCHED FLANK POSE

DAD HELPING SAMUEL, THREE YEARS OLD, INTO UPSIDE-DOWN TREE, ADHO MUKHA VRKSASANA, OR FULL ARM BALANCE

15. JANU SIRSASANA
HEAD TO KNEE POSE, WITH CHIN MUDRA

With one knee bent into *Janu sirsasana* and fingers in *Chin mudra*, which helps the breath to come right from the pelvic floor diaphragm, Will is very relaxed.

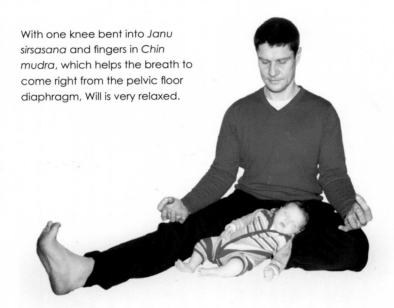

16. Upavistha Konasana
WIDE ANGLE POSE

Still Bella sleeps through it all as Will extends one arm up to release first one hip and then the other (picture at right), feeling that if the hip is moving from the movement of the heel back to the head of the femur then the arm moves up from the lower ribs. (This is where the muscles for the arm have their origin.) Then the movement of the spine forwards comes right from the base.

You do not need to pull yourself from your arms, which would curve your upper back and tighten the shoulders. When you have eased out of one side then the other enough to feel the spine lifted out of the hips, bring your hands down in front (bottom right), spreading down through the fingertips to lengthen up through the arms to broaden the shoulders. Spread the shoulderblades and collarbone so that the spine moves forward and up through shoulders. The spine can then move forward as one from the base right up to the crown.

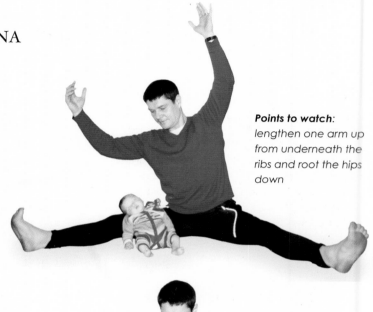

Points to watch: lengthen one arm up from underneath the ribs and root the hips down

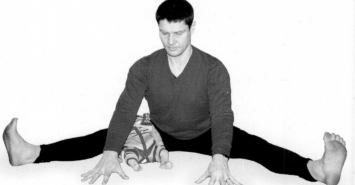

154

BABY SAM IN A PERFECT BADDHA KONASANA

Sam has just naturally put his feet together to make a little Cobbler. No-one put him there. See how straight and alive his spine is! Babies are very free in the hips and alive and naturally lengthened in the spine. As soon as they are put in chairs this starts to go.

If you look carefully at a baby when he or she first crawls, stands and walks you will see first that they are lifted and alive in the sacrum, legs and feet when crawling and that the spine naturally eases out of the sacrum. Then, when they stand, it is all in the legs and feet. They may pull themselves up through their arms and hands but they are grounded and firm in their feet. Then, when they can easily get up and down, they do it entirely from their feet. legs and hips.

Often they are so fascinated by what they have got in their hands, or what they are reaching for. This is what arms and shoulders hands are for: to

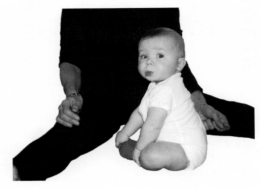

hold and hug. As we get older, we use arms and shoulders to lift us, pushing on armchairs to get up. This makes us slowly lose the use of our legs. Lack of walking and moving from the hips has the same effect, and traps the spine in stiff hips and shoulders.

One of the best movements to give people for this is for them to sit down and then get up again without using the arms at all: first on a chair, then progress to a stool, and then use blocks, gradually reducing their number. See how Will does it, in the inset picture below.

When we can sit on the floor and get up again without using our arms we shall be able to grow old gracefully (as Sri BKS Iyengar says) – keeping the awareness and strength in our legs, just like our children.

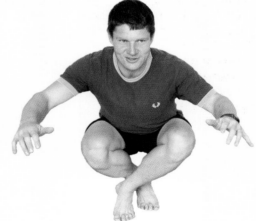

USEFUL ADDRESSES (UK)

GENERAL

Inner Yoga Trust
17 Tilmore Road,
Petersfield, GU32 2HJ
Tel. 01730 261001
www.inneryoga.org.uk

National Childbirth Trust
www.nctpregnancyandbabycare.
com
Tel. 0300 3300 771

Royal College of Midwives
15 Mansfield Road,
London W1G 9NH
Tel. 0207 312 3535
www.rcm.org.uk

UK Department of Health: You can
download THE PREGNANCY BOOK from
www.dh.gov.uk. Search: *pregnancy*

SPECIFIC

Active Birth Centre
www.activebirthcentre.com

Antenatal/postnatal support and
support for parenting: for a list of
local midwifes and health visitors
(Public Health Nurse) seek your
local Health Board

Association for Improvements in the
Maternity Services
www.aims.org.uk

Breastfeeding
– Breastfeeding support: contact
local midwife and public health
nurse as above, or
– Association of Breast Feeding
Mothers Tel. 0870 401 7711
– La Leche League International:
Mothering through breastfeeding
http://www.llli.org
0845 1202918

Sleepless or crying child
You can obtain support through
Cry-sis: http://www.cry-sis.org.uk
Tel. 0845 1228 669

Special needs
The Special Yoga Centre
2a Wrentham Avenue, London
NW10 3HA. Tel. 020 8968 1900
www.specialyoga.org.uk
UK home of The Yoga for the
Special Child programme LLB,
which supports children with
cerebral palsy, Down's syndrome,
autism, epilepsy, attention deficit
disorder and other physical and
developmental difficulties

Support for anyone affected
by the death of a baby
Contact Sands
http://www.uk-sands.org
Tel. 020 7436 5881

EQUIPMENT

Yoga books
Polair Publishing
P O Box 34886
London W8 6YR
www.polairpublishing.co.uk
Distributed in the UK by
www.deep-books.co.uk
and in the USA and Canada by
SCB Distributors

Charts
Charts such as the one mentioned
on p. 110, and other items from
The National Childbirth Trust:
to order ring 0870 112 1120 or visit
www.nctshop.co.uk

Gymnastic balls
(see p. 110) available from www.
simply-yoga.co.uk)

INDEX

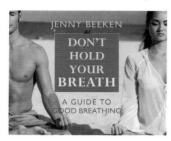
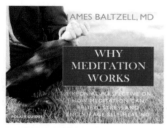
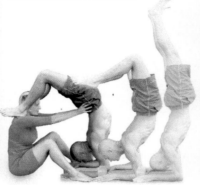
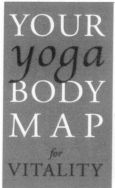
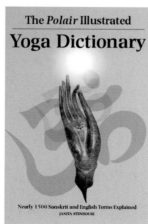
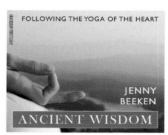
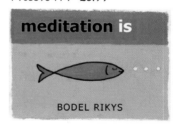